Epilepsy and Schizophrenia: Neurological Disorders

Epilepsy and Schizophrenia: Neurological Disorders

Editor: Noel Day

FOSTER ACADEMICS
www.fosteracademics.com

www.fosteracademics.com

FOSTER ACADEMICS

Cataloging-in-Publication Data

Epilepsy and schizophrenia : neurological disorders / edited by Noel Day.
p. cm.
Includes bibliographical references and index.
ISBN 978-1-63242-541-6
1. Epilepsy. 2. Schizophrenia. 3. Nervous system--Diseases. I. Day, Noel.
RC372 .E65 2018
616.853--dc23

Foster Academics,
118-35 Queens Blvd., Suite 400,
Forest Hills, NY 11375, USA

ISBN 978-1-63242-541-6 (Hardback)

Printed and bound in China.

Contents

Preface VII

Chapter 1 **An Overview of Epilepsy** 1
- Epilepsy 1
- Epilepsy in Children 22

Chapter 2 **Types of Epilepsy** 25
- Abdominal Epilepsy 25
- Idiopathic Generalized Epilepsy 26
- Generalized Epilepsy 35
- Temporal Lobe Epilepsy 36
- Frontal Lobe Epilepsy 45
- Nocturnal Epilepsy 55
- Photosensitive Epilepsy 56
- Post-traumatic Epilepsy 61
- Myoclonic Epilepsy 69

Chapter 3 **Various Epilepsy Syndromes** 72
- Benign Infantile Epilepsy 72
- Benign Familial Infantile Epilepsy 73
- Catamenial Epilepsy 73
- Progressive Myoclonus Epilepsy 78
- Rolandic Epilepsy 80
- Landau-Kleffner Syndrome 84

Chapter 4 **Epileptic Seizure: An Integrated Study** 89
- Epileptic Seizure 89
- Seizure Types 97
- Focal Seizure 101
- Status Epilepticus 117
- Epilepsia Partialis Continua 122

Chapter 5 **Understanding Schizophrenia** ... **125**
- Schizophrenia ... 125
- Paranoid Schizophrenia ... 152
- Disorganized Schizophrenia ... 156
- Pediatric Schizophrenia ... 157
- Mechanisms of Schizophrenia ... 160

Chapter 6 **Schizophrenia: Symptoms, Diagnosis and Management** ... **181**
- Basic Symptoms of Schizophrenia ... 181
- Self-disorder ... 191
- Thought Disorder ... 195
- Delusion ... 198
- Diagnosis of Schizophrenia ... 204
- Causes of Schizophrenia ... 208
- Management of Schizophrenia ... 225

Permissions

Index

Preface

Neurological disorders stem out of the nervous system especially in the spinal cord, nerves and most importantly in the brain. Some of the most common symptoms include confusion, lack of co-ordination, seizures, paralysis, etc. The diseases like schizophrenia and epilepsy are very common neurological diseases. Schizophrenia refers to the disease where the patient has trouble thinking rationally, behaving properly and feeling clearly. Epilepsy refers to violent seizure attacks which result in injuries and many times with broken ribs. This book presents the complex disorders of schizophrenia and epilepsy in the most comprehensible and easy to understand language. The textbook is appropriate for those seeking detailed information in this area.

A short introduction to every chapter is written below to provide an overview of the content of the book:

Chapter 1 - Epilepsy is a set of neurological diseases that cause epileptic seizures. These episodes are caused by synchronous brain activity that are excessive for normal functioning. This chapter will provide an integrated understanding of epilepsy; **Chapter 2 -** Epilepsy can be of various types. They can be classified as being caused by unknown factors, genetic and developmental factors, provoked factors and crytogenic factors. Generalized epilepsy, nocturnal epilepsy, post-traumatic epilepsy, etc. are some of the articles used in this section. The chapter strategically encompasses and incorporates the major components and key concepts of epilepsy, providing a complete understanding; **Chapter 3 -** Epileptic syndromes are analyzed to understand the causes of epilepsy. They also help to identify the suitable medication to be given to treat epilepsy. Epilepsy syndromes are easily detected in children. The topics discussed in the chapter are of great importance to broaden the existing knowledge on epilepsy; **Chapter 4 -** Epileptic seizures occur when the neuronal activity of the brain increases to an abnormal level, causing momentary loss of consciousness and uncontrollable jerking and muscle spasms. Epilepsy causes a paroxysmal depolarizing shift, with brain neurons firing in an uncoordinated manner. The aspects elucidated in this chapter are of vital importance, and provide a better understanding of epilepsy; **Chapter 5 -** Schizophrenia is a mental disorder which affects a person's ability to perceive reality. Symptoms include hearing voices, confusion, paranoia and alienation from the self. The chapter on schizophrenia offers an insightful focus, keeping in mind the complex subject matter; **Chapter 6 -** Schizophrenia is a debilitating mental disorder that causes a variety of symptoms and complications. It is necessary to understand the basic symptoms of schizophrenia so as to assess the development of psychosis in the patient. In order to completely understand schizophrenia, it is necessary to understand the processes related to it. The following chapter elucidates the varied processes and mechanisms associated with this area of study.

I extend my sincere thanks to the publisher for considering me worthy of this task. Finally, I thank my family for being a source of support and help.

Editor

1

An Overview of Epilepsy

Epilepsy is a set of neurological diseases that cause epileptic seizures. These episodes are caused by synchronous brain activity that are excessive for normal functioning. This chapter will provide an integrated understanding of epilepsy.

Epilepsy

Epilepsy is a group of neurological disorders characterized by epileptic seizures. Epileptic seizures are episodes that can vary from brief and nearly undetectable to long periods of vigorous shaking. These episodes can result in physical injuries including occasionally broken bones. In epilepsy, seizures tend to recur and as a rule, have no immediate underlying cause. Isolated seizures that are provoked by a specific cause such as poisoning are not deemed to represent epilepsy. People with epilepsy in some areas of the world experience stigma due to the condition.

The cause of most cases of epilepsy is unknown. Some cases occur as the result of brain injury, stroke, brain tumors, infections of the brain, and birth defects, through a process known as epileptogenesis. Known genetic mutations are directly linked to a small proportion of cases. Epileptic seizures are the result of excessive and abnormal nerve cell activity in the cortex of the brain. The diagnosis involves ruling out other conditions that might cause similar symptoms such as fainting and determining if another cause of seizures is present such as alcohol withdrawal or electrolyte problems. This may be partly done by imaging the brain and performing blood tests. Epilepsy can often be confirmed with an electroencephalogram (EEG), but a normal test does not rule out the condition.

Epilepsy that occurs as a result of other issues may be preventable. Seizures are controllable with medication in about 70% of cases. Inexpensive options are often available. In those whose seizures do not respond to medication, then surgery, neurostimulation, or dietary changes may be considered. Not all cases of epilepsy are lifelong, and many people improve to the point that treatment is no longer needed.

As of 2015 about 39 million people have epilepsy. Nearly 80% of cases occur in the developing world. In 2015 it resulted in 125,000 deaths up from 112,000 deaths in 1990. Epilepsy is more common in older people. In the developed world, onset of new cases occurs most frequently in babies and the elderly. In the developing world onset is more common in older children and young adults, due to differences in the frequency of the underlying causes. About 5–10% of people will have an unprovoked seizure by the age of 80, and the chance of experiencing a second seizure is between 40 and 50%. In many areas of the world those with epilepsy either have restrictions placed on their ability to drive or are not permitted to drive until they are free of seizures for a specific length of time.

Signs and Symptoms

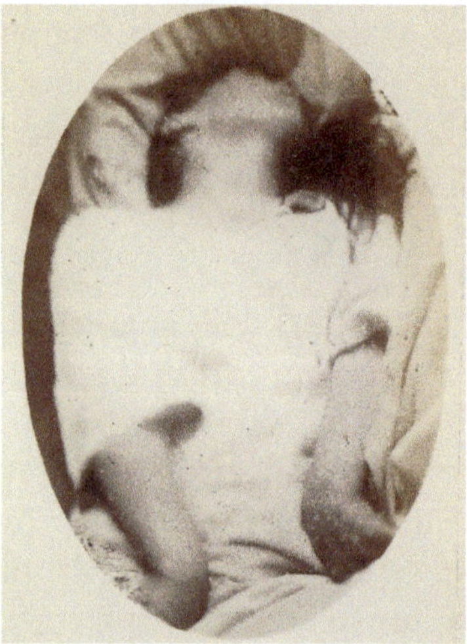

A still image of a generalized seizure

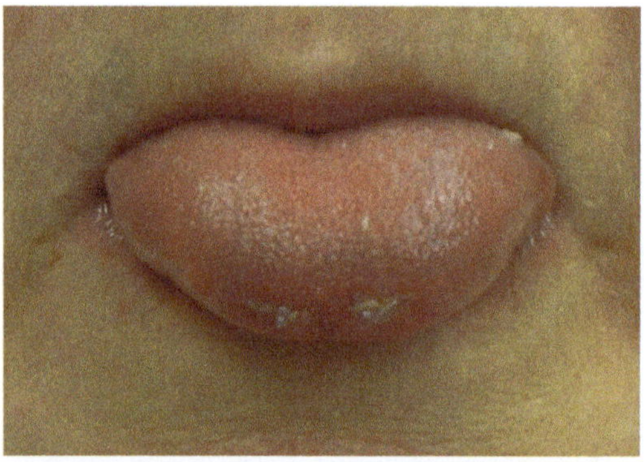

A bite to the tip of the tongue due to a seizure

Epilepsy is characterized by a long-term risk of recurrent seizures. These seizures may present in several ways depending on the part of the brain involved and the person's age.

Seizures

The most common type (60%) of seizures are convulsive. Of these, one-third begin as generalized seizures from the start, affecting both hemispheres of the brain. Two-thirds begin as focal seizures (which affect one hemisphere of the brain) which may then progress to generalized seizures. The remaining 40% of seizures are non-convulsive. An example of this type is the absence seizure, which presents as a decreased level of consciousness and usually lasts about 10 seconds.

Focal seizures are often preceded by certain experiences, known as auras. They include sensory (visual, hearing, or smell), psychic, autonomic, and motor phenomena. Jerking activity may start in a specific muscle group and spread to surrounding muscle groups in which case it is known as a Jacksonian march. Automatisms may occur, which are non-consciously-generated activities and mostly simple repetitive movements like smacking of the lips or more complex activities such as attempts to pick up something.

There are six main types of generalized seizures: tonic-clonic, tonic, clonic, myoclonic, absence, and atonic seizures. They all involve loss of consciousness and typically happen without warning.

Tonic-clonic seizures occur with a contraction of the limbs followed by their extension along with arching of the back which lasts 10–30 seconds (the tonic phase). A cry may be heard due to contraction of the chest muscles, followed by a shaking of the limbs in unison (clonic phase). Tonic seizures produce constant contractions of the muscles. A person often turns blue as breathing is stopped. In clonic seizures there is shaking of the limbs in unison. After the shaking has stopped it may take 10–30 minutes for the person to return to normal; this period is called the "postictal state" or "postictal phase." Loss of bowel or bladder control may occur during a seizure. The tongue may be bitten at either the tip or on the sides during a seizure. In tonic-clonic seizure, bites to the sides are more common. Tongue bites are also relatively common in psychogenic non-epileptic seizures.

Myoclonic seizures involve spasms of muscles in either a few areas or all over. Absence seizures can be subtle with only a slight turn of the head or eye blinking. The person does not fall over and returns to normal right after it ends. Atonic seizures involve the loss of muscle activity for greater than one second. This typically occurs on both sides of the body.

About 6% of those with epilepsy have seizures that are often triggered by specific events and are known as reflex seizures. Those with reflex epilepsy have seizures that are only triggered by specific stimuli. Common triggers include flashing lights and sudden noises. In certain types of epilepsy, seizures happen more often during sleep, and in other types they occur almost only when sleeping.

Postictal

After the active portion of a seizure (the ictal state) there is typically a period of recovery during which there is confusion, referred to as the postictal period before a normal level of consciousness returns. It usually lasts 3 to 15 minutes but may last for hours. Other common symptoms include feeling tired, headache, difficulty speaking, and abnormal behavior. Psychosis after a seizure is relatively common, occurring in 6–10% of people. Often people do not remember what happened during this time. Localized weakness, known as Todd's paralysis, may also occur after a focal seizure. When it occurs it typically lasts for seconds to minutes but may rarely last for a day or two.

Psychosocial

Epilepsy can have adverse effects on social and psychological well-being. These effects may include social isolation, stigmatization, or disability. They may result in lower educational achievement and worse employment outcomes. Learning disabilities are common in those with the condition, and especially among children with epilepsy. The stigma of epilepsy can also affect the families of those with the disorder.

Certain disorders occur more often in people with epilepsy, depending partly on the epilepsy syndrome present. These include depression, anxiety, obsessive–compulsive disorder (OCD), and migraine. Attention deficit hyperactivity disorder affects three to five times more children with epilepsy than children without the condition. ADHD and epilepsy have significant consequences on a child's behavioral, learning, and social development. Epilepsy is also more common in children with autism.

Causes

Epilepsy can have both genetic and acquired causes, with interaction of these factors in many cases. Established acquired causes include serious brain trauma, stroke, tumours and problems in the brain as a result of a previous infection. In about 60% of cases the cause is unknown. Epilepsies caused by genetic, congenital, or developmental conditions are more common among younger people, while brain tumors and strokes are more likely in older people.

Seizures may also occur as a consequence of other health problems; if they occur right around a specific cause, such as a stroke, head injury, toxic ingestion or metabolic problem, they are known as acute symptomatic seizures and are in the broader classification of seizure-related disorders rather than epilepsy itself.

Genetics

Genetics is believed to be involved in the majority of cases, either directly or indirectly. Some epilepsies are due to a single gene defect (1–2%); most are due to the interaction of multiple genes and environmental factors. Each of the single gene defects is rare, with more than 200 in all described. Most genes involved affect ion channels, either directly or indirectly. These include genes for ion channels themselves, enzymes, GABA, and G protein-coupled receptors.

In identical twins, if one is affected there is a 50–60% chance that the other will also be affected. In non-identical twins the risk is 15%. These risks are greater in those with generalized rather than focal seizures. If both twins are affected, most of the time they have the same epileptic syndrome (70–90%). Other close relatives of a person with epilepsy have a risk five times that of the general population. Between 1 and 10% of those with Down syndrome and 90% of those with Angelman syndrome have epilepsy.

Acquired

Epilepsy may occur as a result of a number of other conditions including tumors, strokes, head trauma, previous infections of the central nervous system, genetic abnormalities, and as a result of brain damage around the time of birth. Of those with brain tumors, almost 30% have epilepsy, making them the cause of about 4% of cases. The risk is greatest for tumors in the temporal lobe and those that grow slowly. Other mass lesions such as cerebral cavernous malformations and arteriovenous malformations have risks as high as 40–60%. Of those who have had a stroke, 2–4% develop epilepsy. In the United Kingdom strokes account for 15% of cases and it is believed to be the cause in 30% of the elderly. Between 6 and 20% of epilepsy is believed to be due to head trauma. Mild brain injury increases the risk about two-fold while severe brain injury increases the risk seven-fold. In those who have experienced a high-powered gunshot wound to the head, the risk is about 50%.

Some evidence links epilepsy and coeliac disease and non-celiac gluten sensitivity, while other evidence does not. There appears to be a specific syndrome which includes coeliac disease, epilepsy and calcifications in the brain. A 2012 review estimates that between 1% and 6% of people with epilepsy have CD while 1% of the general population has the condition.

The risk of epilepsy following meningitis is less than 10%; that disease more commonly causes seizures during the infection itself. In herpes simplex encephalitis the risk of a seizure is around 50% with a high risk of epilepsy following (up to 25%). Infection with the pork tapeworm, which can result in neurocysticercosis, is the cause of up to half of epilepsy cases in areas of the world where the parasite is common. Epilepsy may also occur after other brain infections such as cerebral malaria, toxoplasmosis, and toxocariasis. Chronic alcohol use increases the risk of epilepsy: those who drink six units of alcohol per day have a two and a half fold increase in risk. Other risks include Alzheimer's disease, multiple sclerosis, tuberous sclerosis, and autoimmune encephalitis. Getting vaccinated does not increase the risk of epilepsy. Malnutrition is a risk factor seen mostly in the developing world, although it is unclear however if it is a direct cause or an association. People with cerebral palsy have an increased risk of epilepsy, with half of people with spastic quadriplegia and spastic hemiplegia having the disease.

Mechanism

Normally brain electrical activity is non-synchronous. Its activity is regulated by various factors both within the neuron and the cellular environment. Factors within the neuron include the type, number and distribution of ion channels, changes to receptors and changes of gene expression. Factors around the neuron include ion concentrations, synaptic plasticity and regulation of transmitter breakdown by glial cells.

Epilepsy

The exact mechanism of epilepsy is unknown, but a little is known about its cellular and network mechanisms. However, it is unknown under which circumstances the brain shifts into the activity of a seizure with its excessive synchronization.

In epilepsy, the resistance of excitatory neurons to fire during this period is decreased. This may occur due to changes in ion channels or inhibitory neurons not functioning properly. This then results in a specific area from which seizures may develop, known as a "seizure focus". Another mechanism of epilepsy may be the up-regulation of excitatory circuits or down-regulation of inhibitory circuits following an injury to the brain. These secondary epilepsies occur through processes known as epileptogenesis. Failure of the blood–brain barrier may also be a causal mechanism as it would allow substances in the blood to enter the brain.

Seizures

There is evidence that epileptic seizures are usually not a random event. Seizures are often brought on by factors such as stress, alcohol abuse, flickering light, or a lack of sleep, among others. The term seizure threshold is used to indicate the amount of stimulus necessary to bring about a seizure. Seizure threshold is lowered in epilepsy.

In epileptic seizures a group of neurons begin firing in an abnormal, excessive, and synchronized manner. This results in a wave of depolarization known as a paroxysmal depolarizing shift. Normally, after an excitatory neuron fires it becomes more resistant to firing for a period of time. This is due in part to the effect of inhibitory neurons, electrical changes within the excitatory neuron, and the negative effects of adenosine.

Focal seizures begin in one hemisphere of the brain while generalized seizures begin in both hemispheres. Some types of seizures may change brain structure, while others appear to have little effect. Gliosis, neuronal loss, and atrophy of specific areas of the brain are linked to epilepsy but it is unclear if epilepsy causes these changes or if these changes result in epilepsy.

Diagnosis

The diagnosis of epilepsy is typically made based on observation of the seizure onset and the underlying cause. An electroencephalogram (EEG) to look for abnormal patterns of brain waves and neuroimaging (CT scan or MRI) to look at the structure of the brain are also usually part of the workup. While figuring out a specific epileptic syndrome is often attempted, it is not always possible. Video and EEG monitoring may be useful in difficult cases.

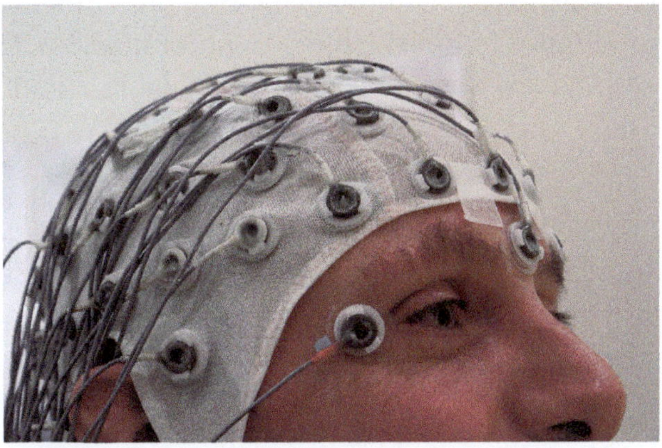

An EEG can aid in locating the focus of the epileptic seizure.

Definition

Epilepsy is a disorder of the brain defined by any of the following conditions:

1. At least two unprovoked (or reflex) seizures occurring greater than 24 hours apart

2. One unprovoked (or reflex) seizure and a probability of further seizures similar to the general recurrence risk (at least 60%) after two unprovoked seizures, occurring over the next 10 years

3. Diagnosis of an epilepsy syndrome

Furthermore, epilepsy is considered to be resolved for individuals who had an age-dependent epilepsy syndrome but are now past that age or those who have remained seizure-free for the last 10 years, with no seizure medicines for the last 5 years.

This 2014 definition of the International League Against Epilepsy is a clarification of the ILAE 2005 conceptual definition, according to which epilepsy is "a disorder of the brain characterized by an enduring predisposition to generate epileptic seizures and by the neurobiologic, cognitive, psychological, and social consequences of this condition. The definition of epilepsy requires the occurrence of at least one epileptic seizure."

It is, therefore, possible to outgrow epilepsy or to undergo treatment that causes epilepsy to be resolved, but with no guarantee that it will not return. In the definition, epilepsy is now called a disease, rather than a disorder. This was a decision of the executive committee of the ILAE, taken because the word "disorder," while perhaps having less stigma than does "disease," also does not express the degree of seriousness that epilepsy deserves.

The definition is practical in nature and is designed for clinical use. In particular, it aims to clarify when an "enduring predisposition" according to the 2005 conceptual definition is present. Researchers, statistically-minded epidemiologists, and other specialized groups may choose to use the older definition or a definition of their own devising. The ILAE considers doing so is perfectly allowable, so long as it is clear what definition is being used.

Classification

In contrast to the classification of seizures which focuses on what happens during a seizure, the classification of epilepsies focuses on the underlying causes. When a person is admitted to hospital after an epileptic seizure the diagnostic workup results preferably in the seizure itself being classified (e.g. tonic-clonic) and in the underlying disease being identified (e.g. hippocampal sclerosis). The name of the diagnosis finally made depends on the available diagnostic results and the applied definitions and classifications (of seizures and epilepsies) and its respective terminology.

The International League Against Epilepsy (ILAE) provided a classification of the epilepsies and epileptic syndromes in 1989 as follows:

1. Localization-related epilepsies and syndromes
    i. Unknown cause (e.g. benign childhood epilepsy with centrotemporal spikes)
    ii. Symptomatic/cryptogenic (e.g. temporal lobe epilepsy)
2. Generalized
    i. Unknown cause (e.g. childhood absence epilepsy)
    ii. Cryptogenic or symptomatic (e.g. Lennox-Gastaut syndrome)
    iii. Symptomatic (e.g. early infantile epileptic encephalopathy with burst suppression)
3. Epilepsies and syndromes undetermined whether focal or generalized
    i. With both generalized and focal seizures (e.g. epilepsy with continuous spike-waves during slow wave sleep)
4. Special syndromes (with situation-related seizures)

This classification was widely accepted but has also been criticized mainly because the underlying causes of epilepsy (which are a major determinant of clinical course and prognosis) were not covered in detail. In 2010 the ILAE Commission for Classification of the Epilepsies addressed this issue and divided epilepsies into three categories (genetic, structural/metabolic, unknown cause) that were refined in their 2011 recommendation into four categories and a number of subcategories reflecting recent technologic and scientific advances.

1. Unknown cause (mostly genetic or presumed genetic origin)
    i. Pure epilepsies due to single gene disorders
    ii. Pure epilepsies with complex inheritance
2. Symptomatic (associated with gross anatomic or pathologic abnormalities)
    i. Mostly genetic or developmental causation
        - Childhood epilepsy syndromes
        - Progressive myoclonic epilepsies
        - Neurocutaneous syndromes
        - Other neurologic single gene disorders
        - Disorders of chromosome function
        - Developmental anomalies of cerebral structure
    ii. Mostly acquired causes
        - Hippocampal sclerosis
        - Perinatal and infantile causes
        - Cerebral trauma, tumor or infection
        - Cerebrovascular disorders
        - Cerebral immunologic disorders
        - Degenerative and other neurologic conditions
3. Provoked (a specific systemic or environmental factor is the predominant cause of the seizures)
    i. Provoking factors
    ii. Reflex epilepsies
4. Crytogenic (presumed symptomatic nature in which the cause has not been identified)

Syndromes

Cases of epilepsy may be organized into epilepsy syndromes by the specific features that are present. These features include the age that seizure begin, the seizure types, EEG findings, among others. Identifying an epilepsy syndrome is useful as it helps determine the underlying causes as well as what anti-seizure medication should be tried.

The ability to categorize a case of epilepsy into a specific syndrome occurs more often with children since the onset of seizures is commonly early. Less serious examples are benign rolandic epilepsy (2.8 per 100,000), childhood absence epilepsy (0.8 per 100,000) and juvenile myoclonic epilepsy (0.7 per 100,000). Severe syndromes with diffuse brain dysfunction caused, at least partly, by some aspect of epilepsy, are also referred to as epileptic encephalopathies. These are associated with frequent seizures that are resistant to treatment and severe cognitive dysfunction, for instance Lennox–Gastaut syndrome and West syndrome. Genetics is believed to play an important role in epilepsies by a number of mechanisms. Simple and complex modes of inheritance have been identified for some of them. However, extensive screening have failed to identify many single gene variants of large effect. More recent exome and genome sequencing studies have begun to reveal a number of de novo gene mutations that are responsible for some epileptic encephalopathies, including CHD2 and SYNGAP1 and DNM1, GABBR2, FASN and RYR3.

Syndromes in which causes are not clearly identified are difficult to match with categories of the current classification of epilepsy. Categorization for these cases was made somewhat arbitrarily. The *idiopathic* (unknown cause) category of the 2011 classification includes syndromes in which the general clinical features and/or age specificity strongly point to a presumed genetic cause. Some childhood epilepsy syndromes are included in the unknown cause category in which the cause is presumed genetic, for instance benign rolandic epilepsy. Others are included in *symptomatic* despite a presumed genetic cause (in at least in some cases), for instance Lennox-Gastaut syndrome. Clinical syndromes in which epilepsy is not the main feature (e.g. Angelman syndrome) were categorized *symptomatic* but it was argued to include these within the category *idiopathic*. Classification of epilepsies and particularly of epilepsy syndromes will change with advances in research.

Tests

An electroencephalogram (EEG) can assist in showing brain activity suggestive of an increased risk of seizures. It is only recommended for those who are likely to have had an epileptic seizure on the basis of symptoms. In the diagnosis of epilepsy, electroencephalography may help distinguish the type of seizure or syndrome present. In children it is typically only needed after a second seizure. It cannot be used to rule out the diagnosis and may be falsely positive in those without the disease. In certain situations it may be useful to perform the EEG while the affected individual is sleeping or sleep deprived.

Diagnostic imaging by CT scan and MRI is recommended after a first non-febrile seizure to detect structural problems in and around the brain. MRI is generally a better imaging test except when bleeding is suspected, for which CT is more sensitive and more easily available. If someone attends the emergency room with a seizure but returns to normal quickly, imaging tests may be done at a later point. If a person has a previous diagnosis of epilepsy with previous imaging, repeating the imaging is usually not needed even if there are subsequent seizures.

For adults, the testing of electrolyte, blood glucose and calcium levels is important to rule out problems with these as causes. An electrocardiogram can rule out problems with the rhythm of the heart. A lumbar puncture may be useful to diagnose a central nervous system infection but is not routinely needed. In children additional tests may be required such as urine biochemistry and blood testing looking for metabolic disorders.

A high blood prolactin level within the first 20 minutes following a seizure may be useful to help confirm an epileptic seizure as opposed to psychogenic non-epileptic seizure. Serum prolactin level is less useful for detecting focal seizures. If it is normal an epileptic seizure is still possible and a serum prolactin does not separate epileptic seizures from syncope. It is not recommended as a routine part of the diagnosis of epilepsy.

Differential Diagnosis

Diagnosis of epilepsy can be difficult. A number of other conditions may present very similar signs and symptoms to seizures, including syncope, hyperventilation, migraines, narcolepsy, panic attacks and psychogenic non-epileptic seizures (PNES). In particular a syncope can be accompanied by a short episode of convulsions. Nocturnal frontal lobe epilepsy, often misdiagnosed as nightmares, was considered to be a parasomnia but later identified to be an epilepsy syndrome. Attacks of the movement disorder paroxysmal dyskinesia may be taken for epileptic seizures. The cause of a drop attack can be, among many others, an atonic seizure.

Children may have behaviors that are easily mistaken for epileptic seizures but are not. These include breath-holding spells, bed wetting, night terrors, tics and shudder attacks. Gastroesophageal reflux may cause arching of the back and twisting of the head to the side in infants, which may be mistaken for tonic-clonic seizures.

Misdiagnosis is frequent (occurring in about 5 to 30% of cases). Different studies showed that in many cases seizure-like attacks in apparent treatment-resistant epilepsy have a cardiovascular cause. Approximately 20% of the people seen at epilepsy clinics have PNES and of those who have PNES about 10% also have epilepsy; separating the two based on the seizure episode alone without further testing is often difficult.

Prevention

While many cases are not preventable, efforts to reduce head injuries, provide good care around the time of birth, and reduce environmental parasites such as the pork tapeworm may be effective. Efforts in one part of Central America to decrease rates of pork tapeworm resulted in a 50% decrease in new cases of epilepsy.

Management

Epilepsy is usually treated with daily medication once a second seizure has occurred, but for those at high risk, medication may be started after the first seizure. In drug-resistant cases different management options may be looked at including a special diet, the implantation of a neurostimulator, or neurosurgery.

First Aid

Rolling a person with an active tonic-clonic seizure onto their side and into the recovery position helps prevent fluids from getting into the lungs. Putting fingers, a bite block or tongue depressor in the mouth is not recommended as it might make the person vomit or result in the rescuer being bitten. Efforts should be taken to prevent further self-injury. Spinal precautions are generally not needed.

If a seizure lasts longer than 5 minutes or if there are more than two seizures in an hour without a return to a normal level of consciousness between them, it is considered a medical emergency known as status epilepticus. This may require medical help to keep the airway open and protected; a nasopharyngeal airway may be useful for this. At home the recommended initial medication for seizure of a long duration is midazolam placed in the mouth. Diazepam may also be used rectally. In hospital, intravenous lorazepam is preferred. If two doses of benzodiazepines are not effective, other medications such as phenytoin are recommended. Convulsive status epilepticus that does not respond to initial treatment typically requires admission to the intensive care unit and treatment with stronger agents such as thiopentone or propofol.

Medications

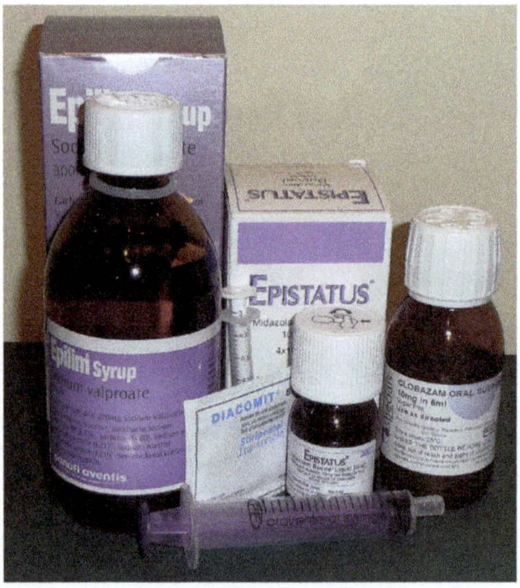

Anticonvulsants

The mainstay treatment of epilepsy is anticonvulsant medications, possibly for the person's entire life. The choice of anticonvulsant is based on seizure type, epilepsy syndrome, other medications used, other health problems, and the person's age and lifestyle. A single medication is recommended initially; if this is not effective, switching to a single other medication is recommended. Two medications at once is recommended only if a single medication does not work. In about half, the first agent is effective; a second single agent helps in about 13% and a third or two agents at the same time may help an additional 4%. About 30% of people continue to have seizures despite anticonvulsant treatment.

There are a number of medications available. Phenytoin, carbamazepine and valproate appear to be equally effective in both focal and generalized seizures. Controlled release carbamazepine appears to work as well as immediate release carbamazepine, and may have fewer side effects. In the United Kingdom, carbamazepine or lamotrigine are recommended as first-line treatment for focal seizures, with levetiracetam and valproate as second-line due to issues of cost and side effects. Valproate is recommended first-line for generalized seizures with lamotrigine being second-line. In those with absence seizures, ethosuximide or valproate are recommended; valproate is particularly effective in myoclonic seizures and tonic or atonic seizures. If seizures are well-controlled on a particular treatment, it is not usually necessary to routinely check the medication levels in the blood.

The least expensive anticonvulsant is phenobarbital at around $5 USD a year. The World Health Organization gives it a first-line recommendation in the developing world and it is commonly used there. Access however may be difficult as some countries label it as a controlled drug.

Adverse effects from medications are reported in 10 to 90% of people, depending on how and from whom the data is collected. Most adverse effects are dose-related and mild. Some examples include mood changes, sleepiness, or an unsteadiness in gait. Certain medications have side effects that are not related to dose such as rashes, liver toxicity, or suppression of the bone marrow. Up to a quarter of people stop treatment due to adverse effects. Some medications are associated with birth defects when used in pregnancy. Many of the common used medications, such as valproate, phenytoin, carbamazepine, phenobarbitol, and gabapentin have been reported to cause increased risk of birth defects, especially when used during the first trimester. Despite this, treatment is often continued once effective, because the risk of untreated epilepsy is believed to be greater than the risk of the medications. Among the antiepileptic medications, levetiracetam and lamotrigine seem to carry the lowest risk of causing birth defects.

Slowly stopping medications may be reasonable in some people who do not have a seizure for two to four years; however, around a third of people have a recurrence, most often during the first six months. Stopping is possible in about 70% of children and 60% of adults.

Surgery

Epilepsy surgery may be an option for people with focal seizures that remain a problem despite other treatments. These other treatments include at least a trial of two or three medications. The goal of surgery is total control of seizures and this may be achieved in 60–70% of cases. Common procedures include cutting out the hippocampus via an anterior temporal lobe resection, removal of tumors, and removing parts of the neocortex. Some procedures such as a corpus callosotomy are attempted in an effort to decrease the number of seizures rather than cure the condition. Following surgery, medications may be slowly withdrawn in many cases.

Neurostimulation may be another option in those who are not candidates for surgery. Three types have been shown to be effective in those who do not respond to medications: vagus nerve stimulation, anterior thalamic stimulation, and closed-loop responsive stimulation.

Diet

A ketogenic diet (high-fat, low-carbohydrate, adequate-protein) appears to decrease the number of seizures and eliminate seizures in some, however further research is necessary. It is a reasonable option in those who have epilepsy that is not improved with medications and for whom surgery is not an option. About 10% stay on the diet for a few years due to issues of effectiveness and tolerability. Side effects include stomach and intestinal problems in 30%, and there are long-term concerns about heart disease. Less radical diets are easier to tolerate and may be effective. It is unclear why this diet works. Exercise has been proposed as possibly useful for preventing seizures with some data to support this claim.

In people with coeliac disease or non-celiac gluten sensitivity and occipital calcifications, a gluten-free diet may decrease the frequency of seizures.

Other

Avoidance therapy consists of minimizing or eliminating triggers. For example, in those who are sensitive to light, using a small television, avoiding video games, or wearing dark glasses may be useful. Operant-based biofeedback based on the EEG waves has some support in those who do not respond to medications. Psychological methods should not, however, be used to replace medications. Some dogs, commonly referred to as seizure dogs, may help during or after a seizure. It is not clear if dogs have the ability to predict seizures before they occur.

Alternative Medicine

Alternative medicine, including acupuncture, psychological interventions, routine vitamins, and yoga, have no reliable evidence to support their use in epilepsy. There is not enough evidence to support the use of cannabis. Melatonin, as of 2016, is insufficiently supported by evidence. The trials were of poor methodological quality and it was not possible to draw any definitive conclusions.

Prognosis

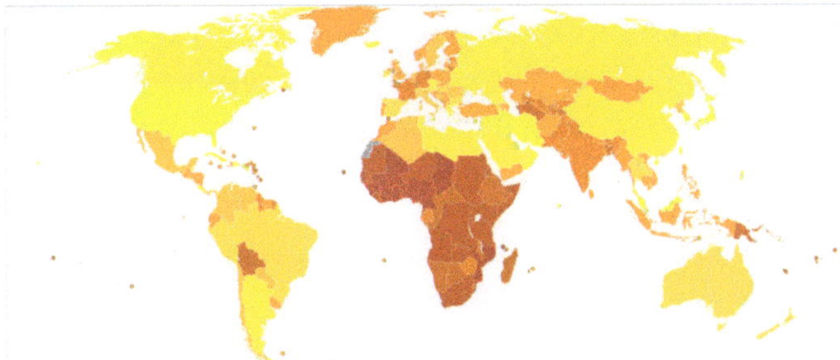

Deaths due to epilepsy per million persons in 2012

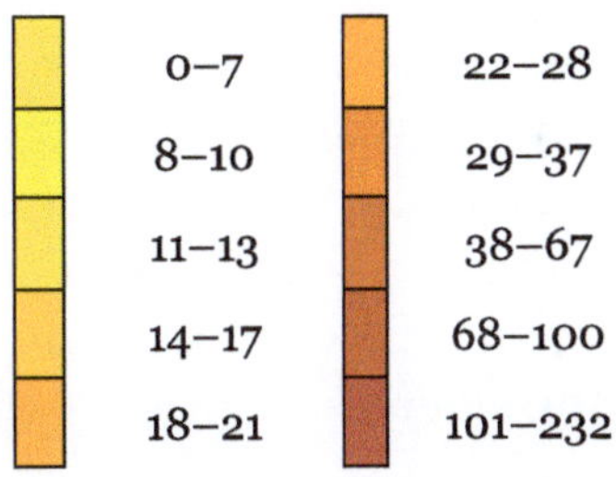

Epilepsy cannot usually be cured, but medication can control seizures effectively in about 70% of cases. Of those with generalized seizures, more than 80% can be well controlled with medications while this is true in only 50% of people with focal seizures. One predictor of long-term outcome is the number of seizures that occur in the first six months. Other factors increasing the risk of a poor outcome include little response to the initial treatment, generalized seizures, a family history of epilepsy, psychiatric problems, and waves on the EEG representing generalized epileptiform activity. In the developing world, 75% of people are either untreated or not appropriately treated. In Africa, 90% do not get treatment. This is partly related to appropriate medications not being available or being too expensive.

Mortality

People with epilepsy are at an increased risk of death. This increase is between 1.6 and 4.1 fold greater than that of the general population and is often related to: the underlying cause of the seizures, status epilepticus, suicide, trauma, and sudden unexpected death in epilepsy (SUDEP). Death from status epilepticus is primarily due to an underlying problem rather than missing doses of medications. The risk of suicide is increased between two and six times in those with epilepsy. The cause of this is unclear. SUDEP appears to be partly related to the frequency of generalized tonic-clonic seizures and accounts for about 15% of epilepsy related deaths. It is unclear how to decrease its risk. The greatest increase in mortality from epilepsy is among the elderly. Those with epilepsy due to an unknown cause have little increased risk. In the United Kingdom, it is estimated that 40–60% of deaths are possibly preventable. In the developing world, many deaths are due to untreated epilepsy leading to falls or status epilepticus.

Epidemiology

Epilepsy is one of the most common serious neurological disorders affecting about 39 million people as of 2015. It affects 1% of the population by age 20 and 3% of the population by age 75. It is more common in males than females with the overall difference being small. Most of those with the disorder (80%) are in the developing world.

The estimated prevalence of active epilepsy (as of 2012) is in the range 3–10 per 1,000, with active epilepsy defined as someone with epilepsy who has had a least one unprovoked seizure in the last five years. Epilepsy begins each year in 40–70 per 100,000 in developed countries and 80–140 per 100,000 in developing countries. Poverty is a risk and includes both being from a poor country and being poor relative to others within one's country. In the developed world epilepsy most commonly starts either in the young or in the old. In the developing world its onset is more common in older children and young adults due to the higher rates of trauma and infectious diseases. In developed countries the number of cases a year has decreased in children and increased among the elderly between the 1970s and 2003. This has been attributed partly to better survival following strokes in the elderly.

History

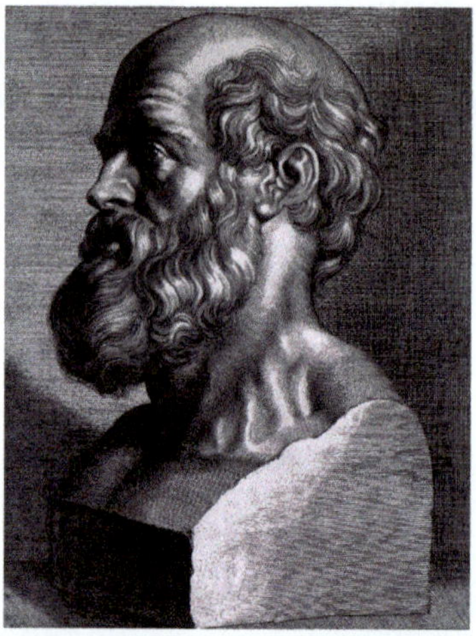

Hippocrates, 17th century engraving by Peter Paul Rubens of an antique bust.

The oldest medical records show that epilepsy has been affecting people at least since the beginning of recorded history. Throughout ancient history, the disease was thought to be a spiritual condition. The world's oldest description of an epileptic seizure comes from a text in Akkadian (a language used in ancient Mesopotamia) and was written around 2000 BC. The person described in the text was diagnosed as being under the influence of a Moon god, and underwent an exorcism. Epileptic seizures are listed in the Code of Hammurabi (c. 1790 BC) as reason for which a purchased slave may be returned for a refund, and the Edwin Smith Papyrus (c. 1700 BC) describes cases of individuals with epileptic convulsions.

The oldest known detailed record of the disease itself is in the *Sakikku*, a Babylonian cuneiform medical text from 1067–1046 BC. This text gives signs and symptoms, details treatment and likely outcomes, and describes many features of the different seizure types. As the Babylonians had no biomedical understanding of the nature of disease, they attributed the seizures to possession by evil spirits and called for treating the condition through spiritual means. Around 900 BC, Punarvasu Atreya described epilepsy as loss of consciousness; this definition was carried forward into the Ayurvedic text of Charaka Samhita (about 400 BC).

The ancient Greeks had contradictory views of the disease. They thought of epilepsy as a form of spiritual possession, but also associated the condition with genius and the divine. One of the names they gave to it was the *sacred disease*. Epilepsy appears within Greek mythology: it is associated with the Moon goddesses Selene and Artemis, who afflicted those who upset them. The Greeks thought that important figures such as Julius Caesar and Hercules had the disease. The notable exception to this divine and spiritual view was that of the school of Hippocrates. In the fifth century BC, Hippocrates rejected the idea that the disease was caused by spirits. In his landmark work *On the Sacred Disease*, he proposed that epilepsy was not divine in origin and instead was a medically treatable problem originating in the brain. He accused those of attributing a sacred cause to the disease of spreading ignorance through a belief in superstitious magic. Hippocrates proposed that heredity was important as a cause, described worse outcomes if the disease presents at an early age, and made note of the physical characteristics as well as the social shame associated with it. Instead of referring to it as the *sacred disease*, he used the term *great disease*, giving rise to the modern term *grand mal*, used for tonic–clonic seizures. Despite his work detailing the physical origins of the disease, his view was not accepted at the time. Evil spirits continued to be blamed until at least the 17th century.

In Ancient Rome people did not eat or drink with the same pottery as that used by someone who was affected. People of the time would spit on their chest believing that this would keep the problem from affected them. According to Apuleius and other ancient physicians, in order detect epilepsy it was common to light a piece of *gagates*, whose smoke would trigger the seizure. Occasionally a spinning potter's wheel was used, perhaps a reference to photosensitive epilepsy.

In most cultures, persons with epilepsy have been stigmatized, shunned, or even imprisoned; in the Salpêtrière, the birthplace of modern neurology, Jean-Martin Charcot found people with epilepsy side-by-side with the mentally ill, those with chronic syphilis, and the criminally insane. In ancient Rome, epilepsy was known as the *morbus comitialis* ('disease of the assembly hall') and was seen as a curse from the gods. In northern Italy, epilepsy was once traditionally known as Saint Valentine's malady.

In the mid-1800s, the first effective anti-seizure medication, bromide, was introduced.

The first modern treatment, phenobarbital, was developed in 1912, with phenytoin coming into use in 1938.

Stigma

Stigma is commonly experienced, around the world, by those with epilepsy. It can affect people economically, socially and culturally. In India and China, epilepsy may be used as justification to deny marriage. People in some areas still believe those with epilepsy to be cursed. In Tanzania, as in other parts of Africa, epilepsy is associated with possession by evil spirits, witchcraft, or poisoning and is believed by many to be contagious, for which there is no evidence. Before 1970 the United Kingdom had laws which prevented people with epilepsy from marrying. The stigma may result in some people with epilepsy denying that they have ever had seizures.

Economics

Seizures result in direct economic costs of about one billion dollars in the United States. Epilepsy resulted in economic costs in Europe of around 15.5 billion Euros in 2004. In India epilepsy is estimated to result in costs of 1.7 billion USD or 0.5% of the GDP. It is the cause of about 1% of emergency department visits (2% for emergency departments for children) in the United States.

Vehicles

Those with epilepsy are at about twice the risk of being involved in a motor vehicular collision and thus in many areas of the world are not allowed to drive or only able to drive if certain conditions are met. In some places physicians are required by law to report if a person has had a seizure to the licensing body while in others the requirement is only that they encourage the person in question to report it themselves. Countries that require physician reporting include Sweden, Austria, Denmark and Spain. Countries that require the individual to report include the UK and New Zealand and the physician may report if they believe the individual has not already. In Canada, the United States and Australia the requirements around reporting vary by province or state. If seizures are well controlled most feel allowing driving is reasonable. The amount of time a person must be free from seizures before they can drive varies by country. Many countries require one to three years without seizures. In the United States the time needed without a seizure is determined by each state and is between three months and one year.

Those with epilepsy or seizures are typically denied a pilot license. In Canada if an individual has had no more than one seizure, they may be considered after five years for a limited license if all other testing is normal. Those with febrile seizures and drug related seizures may also be considered. In the United States, the Federal Aviation Administration does not allow those with epilepsy to get a commercial pilot license. Rarely, exceptions can be made for persons who have had an isolated seizure or febrile seizures and have remained free of seizures into adulthood without medication. In the United Kingdom, a full national private pilot license requires the same standards as a professional driver's license. This requires a period of ten years without seizures while off medications. Those who do not meet this requirement may acquire a restricted license if free from seizures for five years.

Support Organizations

There are organizations that provide support for people and families affected by epilepsy. The *Out of the Shadows* campaign, a joint effort by the World Health Organization, the International League Against Epilepsy and the International Bureau for Epilepsy, provides help internationally. The Joint Epilepsy Council serves the UK and Ireland. In the United States, the Epilepsy Foundation is a national organization that works to increase the acceptance of those with the disease, their ability to function in society and to promote research for a cure. The Epilepsy Foundation, some hospitals, and some individuals also run support groups in the United States.

Other Animals

Epilepsy occurs in a number of other animals including dogs and cats and is the most common brain disorder in dogs. It is typically treated with anticonvulsants such as phenobarbital or bromide in dogs and phenobarbital in cats. Imepitoin is also used in dogs. While generalized seizures in horses are fairly easy to diagnose, it may be more difficult in non-generalized seizures and EEGs may be useful.

Sudden Unexpected Death in Epilepsy

Sudden unexpected death in epilepsy (SUDEP) is a fatal complication of epilepsy. It is defined as the sudden and unexpected, non-traumatic and non-drowning death of a person with epilepsy, without a toxicological or anatomical cause of death detected during the post-mortem examination.

While the mechanisms underlying SUDEP are still poorly understood, it is possibly the most common cause of death as a result of complications from epilepsy, accounting for between 7.5 and 17% of all epilepsy-related deaths and 50% of all deaths in refractory epilepsy. The causes of SUDEP seem to be multifactorial and include respiratory, cardiac and cerebral factors, as well as the severity of epilepsy and seizures. Proposed pathophysiological mechanisms include seizure-induced cardiac and respiratory arrests.

SUDEP occurs in about 1 in 1,000 adults and 1 in 4,500 children with epilepsy a year. Rates of death as a result of prolonged seizures (status epilepticus) are not classified as SUDEP.

Risk Factors

Consistent risk factors include:

- Severity of seizures, increased refractoriness of epilepsy and presence of generalized tonic-clonic seizures: the most consistent risk factor is an increased frequency of tonic–clonic seizures.
- Poor compliance. Lack of therapeutic levels of anti-epileptic drugs, non-adherence to treatment regimens, and frequent changes in regimens are risk factors for sudden death.
- Young age, and early age of seizures onset.
- Male gender
- Poly-therapy of epilepsy. It remains unclear whether this is an independent risk factor or a surrogate marker for severity of epilepsy.
- Being asleep during a seizure is likely to favour SUDEP occurrence.

Mechanism

The mechanisms underlying SUDEP are not well understood but probably involve several pathophysiological mechanisms and circumstances. The most commonly involved are seizure-induced hypoventilation and cardiac arrhythmias but different mechanisms may be involved in different individuals, and more than one mechanism may be involved in any one individual.

- Cardiac factors: cardiac arrhythmias and other cardiac events are known to be involved in some cases of SUDEP. Such arrhythmias are defined as ictal arrhythmias and include the ictal asystole which is a rare occurrence mostly in people that have temporal lobe epilepsy.
- Respiratory factors: impaired respiration and seizure induced pulmonary dysfunction as well as central apnea as a result of brain-stem respiratory centers suppression are known to play a role in some cases of SUDEP.
- Cerebral and autonomic nervous system dysregulation: cardiac arrhythmia and respiratory failure as a result of seizure related changes to brain function and dysfunction of the autonomic nervous system have been described in cases of SUDEP. These include cases of post-ictal generalized EEG suppression described as *cerebral shutdown*, but its significance remains unclear.
- Genetic factors: mutations in several genes have been associated with an increased susceptibility to SUDEP. Over 33% of these are related to mutations which lead to increased susceptibility for arrhythmia. Genes involved include

the hyperpolarization-activated cyclic nucleotide-gated channels genes (HCN1, HCN2, HCN3, and HCN4).

- Anti epileptic drugs: most evidence suggests that antiepileptic drugs are not associated with an increased risk for SUDEP, but rather reduce its incidence. Some studies however indicate that some antiepileptic drugs such as lamotrigine and carbamazepine, may increase the risk of SUDEP in certain individuals. It is unclear if this is because of the potential cardio-respiratory adverse effects such as lengthening of the QT interval and reduction of heart rate known to be associated with these drugs under certain circumstances, or because a high drug dosage could be a surrogate marker for poor seizure control.
- Vagal nerve stimulation: concerns have been raised that vagal nerve stimulation may induce bradycardia or cardiac arrest, and may exacerbate sleep apnoea common in people with epilepsy.

Management

The lack of generally recognized clinical recommendations available are a reflection of the dearth of data on the effectiveness of any particular clinical strategy, but on the basis of present evidence, the following may be relevant:

- Epileptic seizure control with the appropriate use of medication and lifestyle counseling is the focus of prevention.
- Reduction of stress, participation in physical exercises, and night supervision might minimize the risk of SUDEP.
- Knowledge of how to perform the appropriate first-aid responses to seizure by persons who live with epileptic people may prevent death.
- People associated with arrhythmias during seizures should be submitted to extensive cardiac investigation with a view to determining the indication for on-demand cardiac pacing.
- Successful epilepsy surgery may reduce the risk of SUDEP, but this depends on the outcome in terms of seizure control.
- The use of anti suffocation pillows have been advocated by some practitioners to improve respiration while sleeping, but their effectiveness remain unproven because experimental studies are lacking.
- Providing information to individuals and relatives about SUDEP is beneficial.

Epidemiology

- Approximately 50,000 people die each year in the USA from status epilepticus (prolonged seizures), SUDEP, and other seizure-related causes. SUDEP accounts for 8-17% of deaths in people with epilepsy.

- The risk of sudden death in young adults with epilepsy is increased 24-fold compared to the general population.
- SUDEP is the number one cause of epilepsy related death in people with pharmaco-resistant epilepsy.
- Children with epilepsy have a cumulative risk of dying suddenly of 7% within 40 years.
- In children, SUDEP accounts for 34% of all sudden deaths.

Epilepsy in Children

Epilepsy affects all ages groups. But for children, a variety of issues exist that can affect one's childhood.

Some epilepsy ends after childhood. Some forms of epilepsy are associated only with conditions of childhood that cease once a child grows up. Approximately 70% of children who have epilepsy during their childhood eventually outgrow it. There are also some seizures, such as febrile seizures, that are one-time occurrences during childhood, and they do not result in permanent epilepsy.

Effects

Education

Epilepsy can affect a child's education, thereby leading to trouble learning and lower grades. While many children are capable of functioning in a normal classroom environment, many end up in special education.

The child may be forced to miss a lot of school due to seizures. The seizures can impair a child's ability to memorize learning materials.

Tonic-clonic seizures can have a serious impact on education due to the memory loss they cause, and the time needed to recover following the seizure causing there to be missed time in school.

Absence seizures can have a high negative impact on a child's education. As they are less obvious than tonic-clonic seizures, they can occur many times within a single day, thereby resulting in the child's ability to learn being impaired, and leading to low grades.

When seizures are controlled by a medication, many anticonvulsants have side effects that include drowsiness, thereby also impacting a child's education.

The high school graduation rate has been reported at 64%, compared with an overall national average of 82%.

Social

The social stigma can stand in the way, as the child is more prone to bullying.

Many children with epilepsy are overprotected by their parents, who do put restrictions on them in the name of safety, requiring more adult supervision than other children, and not allowing them to participate in certain activities normal to the age group, such as sports. It is a subject of debate if a child with controlled seizures needs additional protection or restrictions, or if the benefits outweigh the losses a child would face.

Causes

The causes of epilepsy in childhood vary. In about ⅔ of cases, it is unknown.

- Unknown 67.6%
- Congenital 20%
- Trauma 4.7%
- Infection 4%
- Stroke 1.5%
- Tumor 1.5%
- Degenerative .7%

Treatment

Most children who develop epilepsy are treated conventionally with anticonvulsants. In about 70% of cases of childhood epilepsy, medication can completely control seizures.

Medicating a child is not always easy. Many pills are made only to be swallowed, which can be difficult for a child. For some medications, chewable versions do exist.

The ketogenic diet is used to treat children who have not responded successfully to other treatments. This diet is low in carbohydrates, adequate in protein and high in fat. It has proven successful in two thirds of epilepsy cases.

In some cases, severe epilepsy is treated with the hemispherectomy, a drastic surgical procedure in which part or all of one of the hemispheres of the brain is removed.

References

- Ryvlin, P; Nashef, L; Tomson, T (May 2013). "Prevention of sudden unexpected death in epilepsy: a realistic goal?". Epilepsia. 54 Suppl 2: 23–8. PMID 23646967. doi:10.1111/epi.12180
- Butler, C (1 March 2005). "Neurological syndromes which can be mistaken for psychiatric conditions". Journal of Neurology, Neurosurgery & Psychiatry. 76 (suppl_1): i31–i38. doi:10.1136/jnnp.2004.060459
- Shorvon, S; Tomson, T (Dec 10, 2011). "Sudden unexpected death in epilepsy.". Lancet. 378 (9808): 2028–38. PMID 21737136. doi:10.1016/S0140-6736(11)60176-1
- Devinsky, Orrin (10 November 2011). "Sudden, Unexpected Death in Epilepsy". New England Journal of Medicine. 365 (19): 1801–1811. doi:10.1056/NEJMra1010481
- Hesdorffer, DC; Tomson, T (Feb 2013). "Sudden unexpected death in epilepsy. Potential role of antiepileptic drugs.". CNS Drugs. 27 (2): 113–9. PMID 23109241. doi:10.1007/s40263-012-0006-1

2

Types of Epilepsy

Epilepsy can be of various types. They can be classified as being caused by unknown factors, genetic and developmental factors, provoked factors and crytogenic factors. Generalized epilepsy, nocturnal epilepsy, post-traumatic epilepsy, etc. are some of the articles used in this section. The chapter strategically encompasses and incorporates the major components and key concepts of epilepsy, providing a complete understanding.

Abdominal Epilepsy

Abdominal epilepsy, also known as autonomic epilepsy, is a rare condition most frequently found in children, consisting of gastrointestinal (GI) disturbances caused by epileptiform seizure activity.

It has been described as a type of temporal lobe epilepsy. Responsiveness to anticonvulsants can aid in the diagnosis.

Most published medical literature dealing with abdominal epilepsy is in the form of individual case reports. A 2005 review article found a total of 36 cases described in the medical literature.

Symptoms

The most common symptom of abdominal epilepsy is abdominal pain followed by uncontrollable vomiting, usually preceded by lethargy. Symptoms also include generalized tonic-clonic seizures followed by sleep, confusion, and unresponsiveness.

Cause

It is unknown as to what causes abdominal epilepsy. While a causal relationship between seizure activity and the GI symptoms has not been proven, the GI symptoms cannot be explained by other pathophysiological mechanisms, and are seen to improve upon anticonvulsant treatment. Because the condition is so rare, no high-quality studies exist. There have been too few reported cases to identify risk factors, genetic factors, or other potential causes.

Diagnosis

Criteria for diagnosis of abdominal epilepsy includes frequent periodic abdominal symptoms, an abnormal electroencephalogram (EEG) and significant improvement of gastrointestinal symptoms after taking anti-seizure medication. Medical testing for diagnosis can be completed using MRI scans of the brain, CT scans and ultrasounds of the abdomen, endoscopy of the gastrointestinal tract, and blood tests.

Treatment

Like other forms of epilepsy, abdominal epilepsy is treated with anticonvulsant drugs, such as Dilantin (phenytoin). Since no controlled studies exist, however, other drugs may be equally effective.

History

Trousseau is commonly credited as being the first to describe the condition in 1868 in a boy with paroxysmal GI symptoms culminating in grand mal epileptic seizure. The first account of abdominal epilepsy supported by EEG tracings came in 1944 in an article by M.T. Moore, followed by subsequent case reports from the same group.

Idiopathic Generalized Epilepsy

Idiopathic generalized epilepsy (IGE) is a group of epileptic disorders that are believed to have a strong underlying genetic basis. Patients with an IGE subtype are typically otherwise normal and have no structural brain abnormalities. People also often have a family history of epilepsy and seem to have a genetically predisposed risk of seizures. IGE tends to manifest itself between early childhood and adolescence although it can be eventually diagnosed later. The genetic cause of some IGE types is known, though inheritance does not always follow a simple monogenic mechanism.

Types

Benign Myoclonic Epilepsy in Infancy

This form of epilepsy is very rare, representing less than 1% of cases, and is twice as prevalent in boys compared to girls. Age of seizure onset is between 5 months and 5 years of age. Children with this disorder often present with head drops and brief arm jerks. Although there is believed to be a genetic basis for this disorder, no genetic linkage has been shown.

Generalized Epilepsy with Febrile Seizures Plus

Generalized epilepsy with febrile seizures plus (GEFS+) is an umbrella for many other syndromes that share causative genes. Patients experience febrile seizures early in childhood and grow to experience other types of seizures later in life. Known causative genes for GEFS+ are the sodium channel α subunit genes SCN1A and SCN2A and the β subunit gene SCN1B. Mutations in the $GABA_A$ receptor γ subunit GABRG1 are also causative for this disorder.

Epilepsy with Myoclonic Absences

This rare epilepsy has a wide age range of presentation (from the first year of life through the early teens). This epilepsy is characterized by absence seizures concurrent with myoclonic jerks, typically occurring several times daily. The genetics of this disorder have not been delineated. Seizures from this disorder often cease within 5 years.

Epilepsy with Myoclonic-astatic Seizures

Originally called Doose syndrome, epilepsy with myoclonic-astatic seizures accounts for ~2% of childhood epilepsies. Children with this disorder have incredibly brief (<100ms) myoclonic jerks followed by equally brief loss of muscle tone, sometimes resulting in dangerous falls. Some patients have much longer lasting seizures of this type. Many patients with this disorder also have absence seizures. This is believed to be a polygenic disorder.

Childhood Absence Epilepsy

Also known as pyknolepsy, childhood absence epilepsy (CAE) represents up to 10% of all childhood epilepsies. It first manifests in childhood between the ages of 4 and 8 as brief periods of unconsciousness (absence). Mutations in the calcium channel α subunit encoding gene CACNA1H and the GABA receptor γ subunit encoding gene GABRG2 yield susceptibility for CAE.

Juvenile Absence Epilepsy

Juvenile absence epilepsy is similar to CAE but has an onset between ages 9 and 13. Other differences are that patients with this disorder have less frequent but longer absence seizures than those with CAE. There are a number of possible genetic loci for this disorder, though no causative genes have been demonstrated.

Juvenile Myoclonic Epilepsy

Also known as Janz syndrome, juvenile myoclonic epilepsy (JME) is a common form of epilepsy, accounting for ~10% of all cases and ~25% of cases of idiopathic generalized epilepsies. Many children with CAE go onto to develop JME. JME first presents between the ages of 12 and 18 with prominent myoclonic seizures. These seizures tend to occur early in the morning. Patients with JME may also have generalized tonic-clonic seizures and absence seizures. Linkage of this disorder has been shown to mutations in the genes GABRA1, CACNB4, CLCN2, GABRD2, EFHC1, and EFHC2.

Epilepsy with Generalized Tonic-clonic Seizures Only

This type of IGE can present at almost any age and is poorly characterized. Because of its loose definition, it is impossible to supply an accurate estimate of its prevalence. As implied by its name, patients with this disorder present only with tonic-clonic seizures.

Childhood Absence Epilepsy

Childhood absence epilepsy (CAE), also known as pyknolepsy, is an idiopathic generalized epilepsy which occurs in otherwise normal children. The age of onset is between 4–10 years with peak age between 5–7 years. Children have absence seizures which although brief (~4–20 seconds), they occur frequently, sometimes in the hundreds per day. The absence seizures of CAE involve abrupt and severe impairment of consciousness. Mild automatisms are frequent, but major motor involvement early in the course excludes this diagnosis. The EEG demonstrates characteristic "typical 3Hz spike-wave" discharges. Prognosis is excellent in well-defined cases of CAE with most patients "growing out" of their epilepsy.

Causes

CAE is a complex polygenic disorder. Particularly in the Han Chinese population there is association between mutations in CACNA1H and CAE. These mutations cause increased channel activity and associated increased neuronal excitability. Seizures are believed to originate in the thalamus, where there is an abundance of T-type calcium channels such as those encoded by CACNA1H.

Pathophysiology

There are currently 20 mutations in CACNA1H associated with CAE. These mutations are likely not wholly causative and should instead be thought of as giving susceptibility. This is particularly true since some groups have found no connection between CAE and CACNA1H mutations. Many of the CACNA1H mutations have a measurable effect on channel kinetics, including activation time constant and voltage dependence, deactivation time constant, and inactivation time constant and voltage dependence. Many of these mutations should lead to neuronal excitability, though others may lead to hypoexcitability. These predictions are due to mathematical modeling and may differ from what will occur in real neurons where other proteins, some of which may interact with CACNA1H, are present.

Along with mutations in CACNA1H, two mutations in the gene encoding a $GABA_A$ receptor γ subunit are also associated with a CAE like phenotype that also overlaps with generalized epilepsy with febrile seizures plus type-3. The first of these, R43Q, abolishes benzodiazepine potentiation of GABA induced currents. The second associated mutation, C588T has not been further characterized.

Diagnosis

Diagnosis is made upon history of absence seizures during early childhood and the observation of ~3 Hz spike-and-wave discharges on an EEG.

Epidemiology

Childhood absence epilepsy is a fairly common disorder with a prevalence of 1 in 1000 people. Few of these people will likely have mutations in CACNA1H or GABRG2 as the prevalence of those in the studies presented is 10% or less.

Juvenile Myoclonic Epilepsy

Juvenile myoclonic epilepsy (JME), also known as Janz syndrome, is a fairly common form of idiopathic generalized epilepsy, representing 5-10% of all epilepsy cases. This disorder typically first manifests itself between the ages of 12 and 18 with brief episodes of involuntary muscle twitching occurring early in the morning. Most patients also have generalized seizures that affect the entire brain and many also have absence seizures. Genetic studies have demonstrated at least 6 loci for JME, 4 with known causative genes. Most of these genes are ion channels with the one non-ion channel gene having been shown to affect ion channel currents.

Signs and Symptoms

Signs of JME are brief episodes of involuntary muscle twitching occurring early in the morning or shortly before falling asleep. This does not usually result in the person falling, but rather dropping objects. These muscle twitching episodes are more common in the arms than in the legs. Other seizure types such as generalized tonic-clonic and absence seizures can also occur. Patients often report quick jerking movements in the morning that results in knocking over objects such as their morning orange juice. Clusters of myoclonic seizures can lead to absence seizures, and clusters of absence seizures can lead to generalized tonic-clonic seizures. The onset of symptoms is generally around age 10-16 although some patients can present in their 20s or even early 30s. The myoclonic jerks generally precede the generalized tonic-clonic seizures by several months. Some people with the disorder never get generalized tonic-clonic seizures (GTCs). Sleep deprivation is a major factor in triggering GTCs. College students often present with a GTC after "pulling an all-nighter." Patients with JME generally do not have other neurological problems.

Cause

Juvenile myoclonic epilepsy is an inherited genetic syndrome, but the way in which this disorder is inherited is unclear. Frequently (17-49%) those with JME have relatives with a history of epileptic seizures. There is also a higher rate of females showing JME symptoms than males. Almost all cases of JME, however, have an onset in early childhood to puberty.

Diagnosis

Diagnosis is typically made based on patient history. The physical examination should be normal. The primary diagnosis for JME is a good knowledge of patient history and the neurologist's familiarity with the myoclonic jerks, which are the hallmark of the syndrome. Additionally, an electroencephalogram (EEG), will indicate a pattern of waves and spikes associated with the syndrome. The EEG generally shows a very characteristic pattern with generalized 4–6 Hz polyspike and slow wave discharges. These discharges are often provoked by photic stimulation (blinking lights) and sometimes hyperventilation. Both a magnetic resonance imaging scan (MRI) and computed tomography scan (CT scan) should appear normal in JME patients.

Pathophysiology

CACNB4

CACNB4 is a gene that encodes the calcium channel β subunit protein. β subunits are important regulators of calcium channel current amplitude, voltage dependence, and also regulate channel trafficking. The β_4 isoform encoded by CACNB4 is most prevalent in the cerebellum. In mice, a naturally occurring null mutation leads to the "lethargic" phenotype, which is similar to JME. There are at least two mutations in the β_4 subunit associated with JME, C104F and R482X. When wild-type α_{1A} and β_4 subunits are expressed in oocytes they produce large Ba^{2+} currents that inactivate slowly. Incorporation of either of the mutant β_4 subunit into channels instead of wild-type subunits produces currents that are larger by 30-40%. The R482X mutation also increases the rate of fast inactivation of the channel. Since these effects are subtle, it is believed that they are contributory rather than completely causative for JME.

GABRA1

GABRA1 is a gene that encodes for an α subunit of the GABA A receptor protein, which encodes one of the major inhibitory neurotransmitter receptors. There is one known mutation in this gene that is associated with JME, A322D, which is located in the third segment of the protein. Expression of the $\alpha_1\beta_2\gamma_2$ combination of subunits in HEK 293 cells produces 6-fold greater current than similar subunits compositions containing mutant α_1 subunits. The mutation also results in greatly decreased sensitivity in the receptor for activation by GABA. This combination of mutant containing receptors also activates far more slowly than wild-type containing receptors. Although originally not reported to result in altered protein trafficking, more recent study has indicated that the A322D mutation reduced α_1 subunit trafficking to the membrane by >90%. Heterozygous expression of wild-type and mutant subunits produces current approximately 50% the size of wild-type due to this altered trafficking.

CLCN2

The CLCN2 gene encodes a chloride channel protein that is heavily expressed in brain regions inhibited by GABA. It is believed to be important in maintaining a proper chloride reversal potential needed in inhibitory neurotransmission by GABA. There are three known mutations in CLCN2 associated with JME, M200fsX231, 74_117del, and G715E. Neither the M200fsX231 nor the 74_117del mutation yield current when expressed in cells. Since these channels are responsible for the removal of intracellular chloride, these mutations are expected to lead to increased chloride concentrations and, thus, altered chloride reversal potential (E_{Cl}). As chloride is conducted through the normally inhibitory GABA receptors, this alteration in E_{Cl} may lead to either decreased GABAergic currents or GABAergic currents that are actually excitatory. The G715E mutation, on the other hand, produces normal sized currents but has altered voltage dependent activation. For this mutant, activation occurs at more positive potentials compared to wild-type channels. This may cause increased neuronal excitability.

GABRD

GABRD encodes the δ subunit of the GABA receptor, which is a subunit yielding receptors which do not desensitize and are localized outside of the synapse. There are three mutations in this gene associated with JME, E177A, R220C, and R220H, all located in the N-terminus of the protein. The last of these mutations is also present in normal controls. Receptors containing the E177A mutation have greatly decreased current compared to wild-type. This is not the case for the R220C mutation but is similar to the R220H mutation, though to a lesser extent than the E177A mutation. More recent study has found that the E177A mutant also has greatly decreased desensitization compared to wild-type receptors. Receptors containing only E177A or R220H mutants, versus heterozygotes, had significantly decreased surface expression compared to wild-type or heterozygotic receptors. These mutants also have decreased single-channel open times compared to wild-type. It should be noted, however, that these mutations are very rare as causes of JME.

EFHC1

The final known associated gene is EFHC1, which is poorly understood. EFHC1 has three DM10 domains (themselves of unknown function) and an EF hand motif, which is known to bind intracellular calcium. EFHC1 is expressed in many tissues, including the brain, where it is localized to the soma and dendrites of neurons, particularly the hippocampal CA1 region, pyramidal neurons in the cerebral cortex, and Purkinje cells in the cerebellum. There are 5 mutations in EFHC1 associated with JME; D210N, F229L, D253Y, P77T and R221H. The last two mutations were originally detected as a pair in the same individual. EFHC1 seems to be involved in programmed cell death as EFHC1 transfected cells have a higher rate of apoptosis. This rate is decreased by the double mutations P77T + R221H. Wild-type EFHC1 increased the R-type calcium channel currents in transfected cells. This stimulation is decreased by JME associated mutations. Because of this, programmed cell death is decreased and the pruning of unwanted neurons may be hampered. As with some other loci, mutations in EFHC1 is not a common loci for JME. More recently, R221H has been found without P77T in one JME kindred.

Other Loci

There is also evidence linking a gene or genes on chromosome 15 (15q14) as well as the BRD2 gene on chromosome 6 (6p21) to JME. Causative genes in this region, however, have not been shown.

Relation to Other Rare Disorders

Until recently, the medical literature did not indicate a connection among many genetic disorders; however, genetic syndromes and genetic diseases are now being found to be related. As a result of new genetic research, some of these are, in fact, highly related in their root cause despite the widely varying set of medical symptoms that are clinically visible in the disorders. This emerging class of diseases are called ciliopathies. The underlying cause may be a dysfunctional molecular mechanism in the primary cilia structures of the cell organelles, which are present in many cellular types throughout the human body. The cilia defects adversely affect "numerous critical developmental signaling pathways" essential to cellular development and thus offer a plausible hypothesis for the often multi-symptom nature of a large set of syndromes and diseases. Known ciliopathies include primary ciliary dyskinesia, Bardet-Biedl syndrome, polycystic kidney and liver disease, nephronophthisis, Alstrom syndrome, Meckel-Gruber syndrome and some forms of retinal degeneration. It has been suggested that juvenile myoclonic epilepsy may be a ciliopathy.

Management

The most effective anti-epileptic medication for JME is valproic acid (Depakote). Women are often started on alternative medications due to valproic acid's high incidence of fetal malformations. Lamotrigine, levetiracetam, topiramate, and zonisamide are alternative anti-epileptic medications with less frequent incidence of pregnancy related complications, and they are often used first in females of childbearing age. Carbamazepine may aggravate primary generalized seizure disorders such as JME. Treatment is lifelong. Patients should be warned to avoid sleep deprivation.

History

The first citation of JME was made in 1857 when Théodore Herpin described a 13-year-old boy suffering from myoclonic jerks, which progressed to tonic-clonic seizures three months later. In 1957, Janz and Christian published a journal article describing several patients with JME. The name Juvenile Myoclonic Epilepsy was proposed in 1975 and adopted by the International League Against Epilepsy.

Myoclonic Astatic Epilepsy

Myoclonic astatic epilepsy, also known as myoclonic atonic epilepsy or Doose syndrome, is a generalized idiopathic epilepsy. It is characterized by the development of myoclonic seizures and/or myoclonic astatic seizures.

Signs and Symptoms

Tonic–clonic Seizures with repetitive sequences of stiffening and jerking of the extremities.

Myoclonic Seizures with rapid, brief contractions of muscles.

Atonic Seizures with a sudden loss of muscle tone, often resulting in sudden collapse. These are also called drop seizures.

Absence A generalized seizure characterized by staring off and occasionally some orofacial automatisms.

Myoclonic astatic Seizures that involve a myoclonic seizure followed immediately by an atonic seizure. This type of seizure is exclusive to MAE and is one of the defining characteristics of this syndrome.

Tonic Muscle stiffening or rigidity. This seizure is rare in this syndrome.

Onset

The onset of seizures is between the ages of 2 and 5. EEG shows regular and irregular bilaterally synchronous 2- to 3-Hz spike-waves and polyspike patterns with a 4- to 7-Hz background. 84% of affected children show normal development prior to seizures; the remainder show moderate psychomotor retardation mainly affecting speech. Boys (74%) are more often affected than girls (Doose and Baier 1987a).

Prognosis

Epilepsy with myoclonic-astatic seizures has a variable course and outcome. Spontaneous remission with normal development has been observed in a few untreated cases. Complete seizure control can be achieved in about half of the cases with antiepileptic drug treatment (Doose and Baier 1987b; Dulac et al. 1990). In the remainder of cases, the level of intelligence deteriorates and the children become severely intellectually disabled. Other neurologic abnormalities such as ataxia, poor motor function, dysarthria, and poor language development may emerge (Doose 1992b). However, this proportion may not be representative because in this series the data were collected in an institution for children with severe epilepsy.

The outcome is unfavorable if generalized tonic-clonic, tonic, or clonic seizures appear at the onset or occur frequently during the course. Generalized tonic-clonic seizures usually occur during the daytime in this disorder, at least in the early stages. Nocturnal generalized tonic-clonic seizures, which may develop later, are another unfavorable sign. If tonic seizures appear, prognosis is poor.

Status epilepticus with myoclonic, astatic, myoclonic-astatic, or absence seizures is another ominous sign, especially when prolonged or appearing early.

Failure to suppress the EEG abnormalities (4- to 7-Hz rhythms and spike-wave discharges) during therapy and absence of occipital alpha-rhythm with therapy also suggest a poor prognosis (Doose 1992a).

Treatments

The treatment for seizures may include antiepileptic medications, diet, and vagus nerve stimulator.

Medication

Any number of medications may be used to both prevent and treat seizures.

Generally after three medications are tried, different treatment should be considered. It should also be noted that some medications are harmful to those with this syndrome and can increase seizures.

Diet

The ketogenic diet mimics some of the effects of starvation, in which the body first uses up glucose and glycogen before burning stored body fat. In the absence of glucose, the body produces ketones, a chemical by-product of fat metabolism that has been known to inhibit seizures.

A modified version of a popular low-carbohydrate, high-fat diet which is less restrictive than the ketogenic diet.

The low glycemic index treatment (LGIT) is a new dietary therapy currently being studied to treat epilepsy. LGIT attempts to reproduce the positive effects of the ketogenic diet. The treatment allows a more generous intake of carbohydrates than the ketogenic diet, but is restricted to foods that have a low glycemic index, meaning foods that have a relatively low impact on blood-glucose levels. These foods include meats, cheeses, and most vegetables because these foods have a relatively low glycemic index. Foods do not have to be weighed, but instead careful attention must be paid to portion size and balancing the intake of carbohydrates throughout the day with adequate amounts of fats and proteins.

History

Myoclonic-Astatic Epilepsy (MAE) was first described and identified in the late 1960s by Herman Doose as an epilepsy syndrome, hence its original label, Doose Syndrome.

Generalized Epilepsy

Generalized epilepsy, also known as primary generalized epilepsy or idiopathic epilepsy, is a form of epilepsy characterised by generalised seizures with no apparent cause. Generalized seizures, as opposed to partial seizures, are a type of seizure that impairs consciousness and distorts the electrical activity of the whole or a larger portion of the brain (which can be seen, for example, on electroencephalography, EEG).

Generalized epilepsy is *primary* because the epilepsy is the originally diagnosed condition itself, as opposed to *secondary* epilepsy, which occurs as a symptom of a diagnosed condition.

Manifestation

Generalized seizures can be either absence seizures, myoclonic seizures, clonic seizures, tonic-clonic seizures or atonic seizures.

Generalized seizures occur in various seizure syndromes, including myoclonic epilepsy, familial neonatal convulsions, childhood absence epilepsy, absence epilepsy, infantile spasms (West's syndrome), Juvenile Myoclonic Epilepsy and Lennox-Gastaut syndrome.

Prognosis

Most generalized epilepsy starts during childhood. While some patients outgrow their epilepsy during adolescence and no longer need medication, in others, the condition remains for life, thereby requiring lifelong medication and monitoring.

Treatment

Seven anti-epileptic drugs are approved for use in cases of suspected primary generalized epilepsy:

- Felbamate

- Levetiracetam
- Zonisamide
- Topiramate
- Valproate
- Lamotrigine
- Perampanel

Valproate, a relatively old drug, is often considered the first-line treatment. It is highly effective, but its association with fetal malformations when taken in pregnancy limits its use in young women.

All anti-epileptic drugs (including the above) can be used in cases of partial seizures.

Temporal Lobe Epilepsy

Temporal lobe epilepsy (TLE) is a chronic disorder of the nervous system characterized by recurrent, unprovoked focal seizures that originate in the temporal lobe of the brain and last about one or two minutes. TLE is the most common form of epilepsy with focal seizures. People with TLE may experience simple partial seizures that only affect the temporal lobe or complex partial seizures that spread to other regions of the brain.

TLE is usually diagnosed in childhood or by the teenage years. Physicians diagnose TLE by taking a medical history, blood tests, and brain imaging. It can have a number of causes such as head injury, stroke, brain infections, structural lesions in the brain, or brain tumors, or it can be idiopathic and have no apparent cause. The first line of treatment is through anticonvulsant medication. Surgery may be an option for some people, especially when there is an observable abnormality in the brain. Another treatment option is electrical stimulation of the brain through an implantation called the vagus nerve stimulation (VNS) device.

Types

Over forty types of epilepsy are recognized and these are divided into two main seizures: Partial seizure and generalized seizure. Partial seizures account for approximately sixty percent of all adult cases. Temporal lobe epilepsy (TLE) is the single most common form of partial seizure.

The International League Against Epilepsy (ILAE) recognizes two main types of temporal lobe epilepsy: mesial temporal lobe epilepsy (MTLE), arising in the hippocampus, the parahippocampal gyrus and the amygdala which are located in the inner (medial) aspect of the temporal lobe and lateral temporal lobe epilepsy (LTLE), the rarer type, arising in the neocortex at the outer (lateral) surface of the temporal lobe. The seizures of LTLE are characterized by auditory or visual features. Autosomal dominant Lateral Temporal Lobe Epilepsy (ADLTLE) is a rare hereditary condition.

Signs and Symptoms

When a seizure begins in the temporal lobe, its symptoms and the patient's behavior as seen by bystanders, depend on the precise location of its point of origin, its *locus*. In 1981, the ILAE recognized three types of seizures occurring in temporal lobe epilepsy. The classification was based on EEG findings.

Simple Partial Seizures

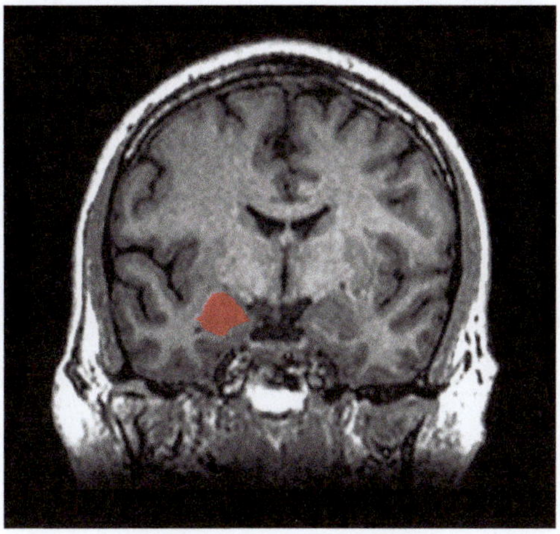

MRI Location Amygdala

Simple partial seizures (SPS) involve small areas of the temporal lobe such as the amygdala and hippocampus. The term "simple" means that the level of consciousness of the patient is not altered during the seizure. In temporal lobe epilepsy, a simple partial seizure usually causes abnormal sensations only.

These may be:

- Mnestic sensations such as déjà vu (a feeling of familiarity), jamais vu (a feeling of unfamiliarity)
- amnesia; or a single memory or set of memories
- A sudden sense of unprovoked fear and anxiety
- Nausea
- Auditory, visual, olfactory, gustatory, or tactile hallucinations.

- Visual distortions such as macropsia and micropsia
- Dissociation or derealisation
- Synesthesia (stimulation of one sense experienced in a second sense) may transpire.
- Dysphoric or euphoric feelings, fear, anger, and other emotions may also occur. Often, the patient cannot describe the sensations.

Olfactory hallucinations often seem indescribable to patients beyond "pleasant" or "unpleasant".

Simple partial seizures may be called "auras" by lay people who mistake them for a warning sign of a subsequent seizure. Instead, the so-called *aura* is actually the *partial* seizure itself. People who only experience simple partial seizures may not recognize what they are, nor seek medical advice about them. A simple partial seizure may or may not progress to any of the seizure types listed below.

Complex Partial Seizures

Complex partial seizures (CPS) are seizures which impair consciousness to some extent: they alter the person's ability to interact normally with their environment. They usually begin with a simple partial seizure, then spread to a larger portion of the temporal lobe, resulting in impaired consciousness. They may include autonomic and psychic features present in simple partial seizures.

Signs may include:

- Motionless staring
- Automatic movements of the hands or mouth
- Confusion and disorientation
- Altered ability to respond to others, unusual speech
- Transient aphasia (losing ability to speak, read, or comprehend spoken word)

These seizures tend to have a warning or aura before they occur, and when they occur they generally tend to last only 1–2 minutes. It is not uncommon for an individual to be tired or confused for up to 15 minutes after a seizure has occurred, although postictal confusion can last for hours or even days. Though they may not seem harmful, due to the fact that the individual does not normally seize, they can be extremely harmful if the individual is left alone around dangerous objects. For example, if a person with complex partial seizures is driving alone, this can cause them to run into the ditch, or worse, cause an accident involving multiple people. With this type, some people do not even realize they are having a seizure and most of the time their memory from right before or after the seizure is wiped. First-aid is only required if there has been an injury or if this is the first time a person has had a seizure.

Secondarily Generalized Tonic-clonic Seizures

Seizures which begin in the temporal lobe, and then spread to involve the whole brain are known as Secondarily Generalized Tonic-Clonic Seizures (SGTCS). The arms, trunk, and legs stiffen (the tonic phase), in either a flexed or extended position, and then jerk (the clonic phase). Secondarily generalized tonic clonic seizures are known in the vernacular as *convulsions* or *grand mal* seizures. The word *grand mal* comes from the French term, meaning *major affliction*.

Postictal Period

There is some period of recovery in which neurological function is altered after each of these seizure types. This is the *postictal state*. The degree and length of postictal impairment directly correlates with the severity of the seizure type. Simple partial seizures often last less than sixty seconds; complex partial seizures may last up to two minutes; and generalized tonic clonic seizures may last up to three minutes. The postictal state in the case of complex partial seizures and generalised tonic clonic seizures may last much longer than the seizure itself.

Because a major function of the temporal lobe is short-term memory, complex partial seizures and generalised tonic clonic seizures may cause amnesia for the period of the seizure. As a result, patients with temporal lobe complex partial seizures and generalised tonic clonic seizures may not remember having had a seizure.

Complications and Prognosis

Depression

Individuals with temporal lobe epilepsy have a higher prevalence of depression than the general population. Although the psychosocial impacts of epilepsy may be causative, there are also links in the phenomenology and neurobiology of TLE and depression.

Memory

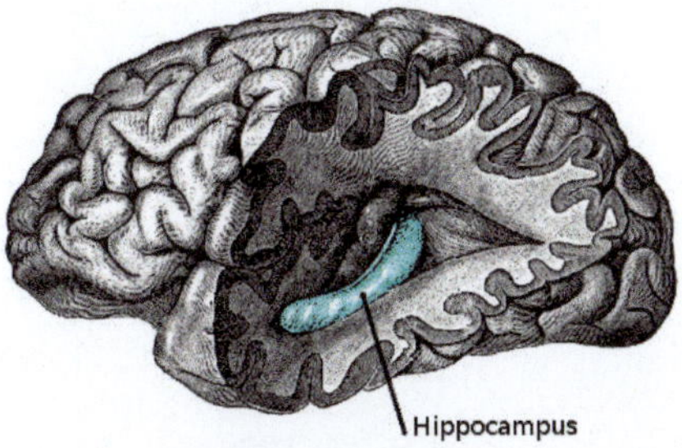

Hippocampus

The temporal lobe and particularly the hippocampus plays an important role in memory processing. Declarative memory (memories which can be consciously recalled) is formed in the area of the hippocampus called the *dentate gyrus*.

Temporal lobe epilepsy is associated with memory disorders and loss of memory. Animal models and clinical studies show that memory loss correlates with temporal lobe neuronal loss in temporal lobe epilepsy. Verbal memory deficit correlates with pyramidal cell loss in TLE. This is more so on the left in verbal memory loss. Neuronal loss on the right is more prominent in non-verbal (visuospatial memory loss).

Childhood Onset

After childhood onset, one third will "grow out" of TLE, finding a lasting remission up to an average of 20 years. The finding of a lesion such as hippocampal sclerosis (a scar in the hippocampus), tumour, or dysplasia, on magnetic resonance imaging (MRI) predicts the intractability of seizures.

Personality

The effect of temporal lobe epilepsy on personality is an historical observation dating to the 1800s. Personality and behavioural change in temporal lobe epilepsy is seen as a chronic condition when it persists for more than three months.

Geschwind syndrome is a behavioural phenomena evident in some people with TLE documented by Norman Geschwind, involving Hypergraphia (overwhelming compulsion to draw or write), Hyperreligiosity (intense religious experiences or interests), Atypical sexuality (normally reduced or asexual), circumstantiality (result of a non-linear thought pattern, talks at length about irrelevant and trivial details).

Diagnosis

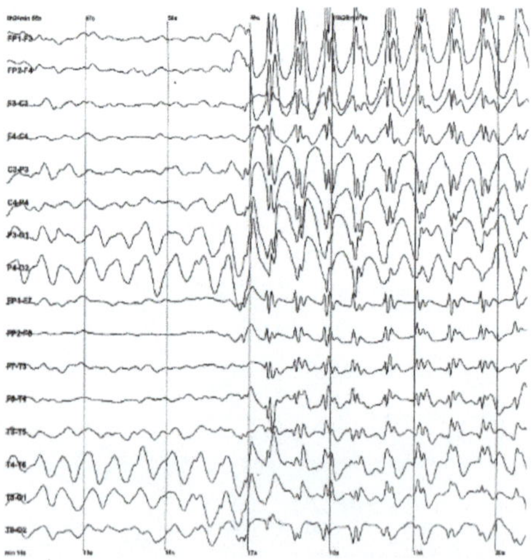

Epileptic spike and wave discharges monitored with EEG

Temporal lobe epilepsy diagnosis can be done via the following methods/exams:

- MRI
- CT scan
- Positron Emission Tomography
- Electroencephalography
- Magnetoencephalography

Differential Diagnosis

Among the DDx to look out for are panic attacks, psychosis spectrum disorders, tardive dyskinesia, and occipital lobe epilepsy (though this is not an exhaustive list)

Causes

The causes of TLE include mesial temporal sclerosis, traumatic brain injury, brain infections, such as encephalitis and meningitis, hypoxic brain injury, stroke, cerebral tumours, and genetic syndromes. Temporal lobe epilepsy is not the result of mental health disorders or fragility of the personality.

Febrile Seizures

Although the theory is controversial, there is a link between febrile seizures (seizures coinciding with episodes of fever in young children) and subsequent temporal lobe epilepsy, at least epidemiologically.

Human Herpes Virus 6

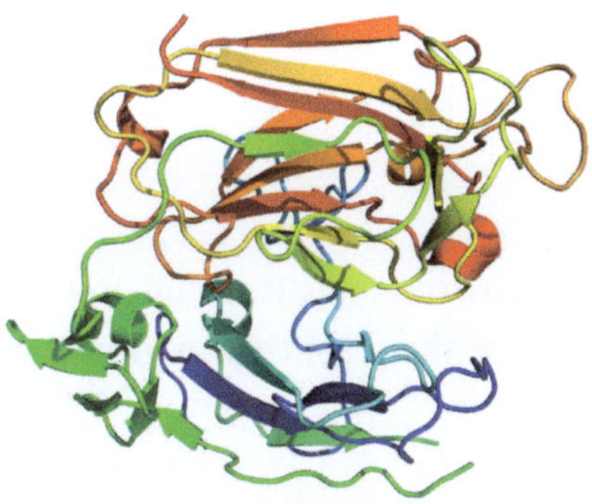

Reelin

In the mid 1980s, human herpesvirus 6 (HHV-6) was suggested as a possible causal link between febrile convulsions and mesial temporal lobe epilepsy. However, although the virus is found in temporal lobe tissue at surgery for TLE, it has not been recognised as a major factor in febrile seizures or TLE.

Reelin

Dispersion of the granule cell layer in the hippocampal dentate gyrus is occasionally seen in temporal lobe epilepsy and has been linked to the downregulation of reelin, a protein that normally keeps the layer compact by containing neuronal migration. It is unknown whether changes in reelin expression play a role in epilepsy.

Pathophysiology

Neuronal Loss

In TLE, there is loss of neurons in region CA1 and CA3 of the hippocampus. There is also damage to mossy cells and inhibitory interneurons in the hilar region of the hippocampus (region IV) and to the granule cells of the dentate gyrus. In animal models, neuronal loss occurs during seizures but in humans, neuronal loss predates the first seizure and does not necessarily continue with seizure activity. The loss of the GABA-mediated inhibitory interneurons may increase the hyperexcitability of neurons of the hippocampus leading to recurrent seizures. According to the "dormant basket cell" hypothesis, mossy cells normally excite basket cells which in turn, inhibit granule cells. Loss of mossy cells lowers the threshold of action potentials of the granule cells.

Granule Cell Dispersion in the Dentate Gyrus

Granule cell dispersion is a type of developmental migration and a pathological change found in the TLE brain which was first described in 1990. The granule cells of the dentate gyrus are tightly packed forming a uniform, laminated layer with no monosynaptic connections. This structure provides a filter for the excitability of neurons.

In TLE, granule cells are lost, the structure is no longer closely packed and there are changes in the orientation of dendrites. These changes may or may not be epileptogenic. For instance, if the dendrites of granule cells reconnect, it may be in a way (through the laminar planes) that allows hyperexcitability. However, not all patients have granule cell dispersion.

Aberrant Mossy Fiber Sprouting

Mossy fibers are the axons of Ponte nuclei cells. They project into the hilum of the dentate gyrus and stratum lucidum in the CA3 region giving input to both excitatory and inhibitory neurons.

In the TLE brain, where granule cells are damaged or lost, axons, the *mossy* fibres, 'sprout' in order to reconnect to other granule cell dendrites. This is an example of *synaptic reorganisation*. This was noted in human tissue in 1974 and in animal models in 1985. In TLE, the sprouting mossy fibres are larger than in the normal brain and their connections may be aberrant. Mossy fibre sprouting continues from one week to two months after injury.

Aberrant mossy fibre sprouting may create excitatory feedback circuits that lead to temporal lobe seizures. This is evident in intracellular recordings. Stimulation of aberrant mossy fibre areas increases the excitatory postsynaptic potential response.

However, aberrant mossy fiber sprouting may inhibit excitatory transmission by synapsing with basket cells which are inhibitory neurons and by releasing GABA and neuropeptide Y which are inhibitory neurotransmitters. Also, in animal models, granule cell hyper-excitability is recorded before aberrant mossy fibre sprouting has occurred.

Treatments

Antiepileptic Drugs

There are many oral medications available for the management of epileptic seizures. They were previously called anticonvulsants. However, this term is misleading because most TLE seizures are, in fact, not *convulsions*. The modern term is *antiepileptic drugs* (AEDs). Nearly all AEDs function by decreasing the excitation of neurons, for example, by blocking fast or slow sodium channels or by modulating calcium channels; or by enhancing the inhibition of neurons, for example by potentiating the effects of inhibitory neurotransmitters like GABA.

In TLE, the most commonly used older AEDs are phenytoin, carbamazepine, primidone, valproate, and phenobarbital. Newer drugs, such as gabapentin, topiramate, levetiracetam, lamotrigine, pregabalin, tiagabine, lacosamide, and zonisamide promise similar effectiveness, with possibly fewer side-effects. Felbamate and vigabatrin are newer AEDs, but can have serious adverse effects so they are not considered first-line treatments.

Up to one third of patients with medial temporal lobe epilepsy will not have adequate seizure control with medication alone. For patients with medial TLE whose seizures remain uncontrolled after trials of several AEDs (that is, the epilepsy is *intractable*), surgical excision of the affected temporal lobe may be considered.

Surgical Interventions

Epilepsy surgery has been performed since the 1860s and doctors have observed that it is highly effective in producing freedom from seizures. However, it was not until 2001 that a scientifically sound study was carried out to examine the effectiveness of temporal lobectomy.

Temporal lobe surgery can be complicated by decreased cognitive function. However, after temporal lobectomy, memory function is supported by the opposite temporal lobe; and recruitment of the frontal lobe. Cognitive rehabilitation may also help.

Other Treatments

If a person is not an optimal candidate for epilepsy surgery, further management options include new (including experimental) antiepileptic drugs, vagus nerve stimulation, and in children, the ketogenic diet. Other avenues of treatment include brain cortex responsive neural stimulators, deep brain stimulation, stereotactic radiosurgery, such as the gamma knife, and stereotactic laser ablation.

Link with Religiosity

The first to record and catalog the abnormal symptoms and signs of TLE was Norman Geschwind. He found a constellation of symptoms that included hypergraphia, hyperreligiosity, collapse, and pedantism, now called *Geschwind syndrome*.

Vilayanur S. Ramachandran explored the neural basis of the hyperreligiosity seen in TLE using the galvanic skin response (GSR), which correlates with emotional arousal, to determine whether the hyperreligiosity seen in TLE was due to an overall heightened emotional state or was specific to religious stimuli. Ramachandran presented two subjects with neutral, sexually arousing and religious words while measuring GSR. Ramachandran was able to show that patients with TLE showed enhanced emotional responses to the religious words, diminished responses to the sexually charged words, and normal responses to the neutral words. This study was presented as an abstract at a neuroscience conference and referenced in Ramachandran's book, *Phantoms in the Brain*, but it has never been published in the peer-reviewed scientific press.

One recent study reported that intrinsic religiosity and religiosity outside of organized religion were higher in patients with epilepsy than in controls. Lower education level, abnormal background EEG activity, and hippocampal sclerosis have been found to be contributing factors for religiosity in Temporal Lobe Epilepsy.

Temporal lobe epilepsy has been suggested as a physical explanation for the revelatory experiences of prominent religious figures such as Abraham, Moses, Jesus, Mohammed, Saint Paul, and Joseph Smith. These experiences are described as complex interactions with their visions, but lacking the stereotypy, amnestic periods, and automatisms or generalized motor events, which are characteristic of TLE. Psychiatric conditions with psychotic spectrum symptoms may be a more plausible physical explanation of these experiences. Pope Pius IX's doctrine of the immaculate conception is thought to have been influenced by his forensically diagnosed partial epilepsy. It has also been suggested that the visions of Joan of Arc were probably an expression of partial epilepsy. More recently, one case history found that a temporal lobe epileptic experienced a vision of God following a temporal lobe seizure, while undergoing EEG monitoring. The patient reported that God had sent him to the world to "bring redemption to the people of Israel". The purported link between TLE and religiosity has inspired work by Michael Persinger and many other researchers in the field of neurotheology, but some have questioned the evidence for a link between temporal lobe epilepsy and religiosity. The novel, *Lying Awake*, by Mark Salzman, deals with topic of temporal lobe epilepsy and religion.

Frontal Lobe Epilepsy

Frontal lobe epilepsy, or FLE, is a neurological disorder that is characterized by brief, recurring seizures that arise in the frontal lobes of the brain, often while the patient is sleeping. It is the second most common type of epilepsy after temporal lobe epilepsy (TLE), and is related to the temporal form by the fact that both forms are characterized by the occurrence of partial (focal) seizures. Partial seizures occurring in the frontal lobes can occur in one of two different forms: either simple partial seizures (that do not affect awareness or memory) or complex partial seizures (that affect awareness or memory either before, during or after a seizure). The symptoms and clinical manifestations of frontal lobe epilepsy can differ depending on which specific area of the frontal lobe is affected.

The onset of a seizure may be hard to detect since the frontal lobes contain and regulate many structures and functions about which relatively little is known. Due to the lack of knowledge surrounding the functions associated with the frontal lobes, seizures occurring in these regions of the brain may produce unusual symptoms which can often be misdiagnosed as a psychiatric disorder, non-epileptic seizure or a sleep disorder.

During the onset of a seizure, the patient may exhibit abnormal body posturing, sensorimotor tics, or other abnormalities in motor skills. In some cases, uncontrollable laughing or crying may occur during a seizure. Afflicted persons may or may not be aware that they are behaving in an abnormal manner, depending on the patient and type of seizure. A brief period of confusion known as a postictal state may sometimes follow a seizure occurring in the frontal lobes. However, these postictal states are often undetectable and generally do not last as long as the periods of confusion following seizures that occur in the temporal lobes.

There are many different causes of frontal lobe epilepsy ranging from genetics to head trauma that result in lesions in the frontal lobes. Although frontal lobe epilepsy is often misdiagnosed, tests such as prolonged EEG monitoring and/or a MRI scan of the frontal lobes can be administered in order to reveal the presence of a tumor or vascular malformation. Unlike most epileptic EEGs, the abnormalities in FLE EEGs precede the physical onset of the seizure and aid in localization of the seizure's origin. Medications such as anti-epileptic drugs can typically control the onset of seizures, however, if medications are ineffective the patient may undergo surgery to have focal areas of the frontal lobe removed.

Signs and Symptoms

Epileptic symptoms are frequently the product of the spread of overactivation occurring within one central foci that travels to lateral brain regions thereby causing an array of symptoms. Due to the massive amount of diversity in both the cognitive and motor functions that occur within the frontal lobes, there is an immense variety in the types of symptoms that can arise from epileptic seizures based on the side and topography of the focal origin. In general these symptoms can range anywhere from asymmetric and abnormal body positioning to repetitive vocal outburts and repetitive jerking movements. The symptoms typically come in short bursts that last less than a minute and often occur while a patient is sleeping. In most cases, a patient will experience a physical or emotional Aura of tingling, numbness or tension prior to a seizure occurring. Fear is associated with temporal and frontal lobe epilepsies, but in FLE the fear is predominantly expressed on the person's face whereas in TLE the fear is subjective and internal, not perceptible to the observer.

Tonic posture and clonic movements are common symptoms among most of the areas of the frontal lobe, therefore the type of seizures associated with frontal lobe epilepsy are commonly called tonic-clonic seizures. Dystonic motor movements are common to both TLE and FLE, but are usually the first symptom in FLE episodes where they are quite brief and do not affect consciousness. The seizures are complex partial, simple partial, secondarily generalized or a combination of the three. These partial seizures are often misdiagnosed as psychogenic seizures. A wide range of more specific symptoms arise when different parts of the frontal cortex are affected.

- Supplementary motor area (SMA)
  - The onset and relief of the seizure are quite abrupt.
  - The tonic posturing in this area is unilateral or asymmetric between the left and right hemispheres. A somatosensory aura frequently precedes many large motor and vocal symptoms and most often the afflicted person is responsive.
  - *Motor symptoms*: Facial grimacing and complex automatisms like kicking and pelvic thrusting
  - *Vocal symptoms*: Laughing, yelling, or speech arrest.
- Primary motor cortex
  - The primary motor cortex has jacksonian seizures that spread to adjacent areas of the lobe which often trigger a second round of seizures originating in another cortical area. The seizures are much simpler than those that originate in the SMA and are usually clonic or myoclonic movements with speech arrest. Some dystonic or contralateral adversive posturing may also be present.
- Medial frontal, cingulate gyrus, orbitofrontal, or frontopolar regions
  - Motor symptoms of seizures in this area are accompanied by emotional feelings and viscerosensory symptoms. Motor and vocal agitation are similar to that of the SMA with short repetitive thrashing, pedaling, thrusting, laughing, screaming and/or crying.
  - This is some of what can cause the misdiagnosis of a psychological disorder.

- Dorsolateral cortex
  - This area does not seem to have many motor symptoms beyond tonic posturing or clonic movements. Contralateral or less commonly ipsilateral head turn and eye deviation are commonly associated with this area as well.
- Operculum
  - Many of the symptoms associated with this area involve the head and digestive tract: swallowing, salivation, mastication and possibly gustatory hallucinations. Preceding the seizure the person is fearful and often has an epigastric aura. There is not much physical movement except clonic facial movements. Speech is often arrested.

Common Misdiagnoses

Episodes that include complex hyperactivity of the proximal portions of the limbs that lead to increased overall motor activity are called hypermotor seizures. When associated with bizarre movements and vocalizations these seizures are often misdiagnosed as pseudoseizures or other episodic movement disorders such as psychogenic movement disorders, familial paroxysmal dystonic choreoathetosis, paroxysmal kinesogenic choreoathetosis, or episodic ataxia type 1. Hypermotor seizure in children are often confused with pavor nocturnus (night terrors). Paroxysmal nocturnal dystonia or hypnogenic paroxysmal dystonia are other names given to describe FLE symptoms but are simply just FLE.

Autosomal Dominant Nocturnal Frontal Lobe Epilepsy (ADNFLE) is the best understood form of frontal lobe epilepsy but is often misdiagnosed as sleep apnea. Both disorders are characterized by awakening during the night which leads to daytime sleepiness. Some symptoms of sleep apnea overlap with those of ADNFLE, such as sudden awakening accompanied by a feeling of choking and on occasion motor activity which makes diagnosis difficult based on symptoms alone. Video surveillance as well as EEG is occasionally needed to differentiate between the two disorders. It has been reported that sleep apnea might be associated with epilepsy which would account for some of the misdiagnoses.

Causes

The origins of frontal lobe seizures range from tumors to head trauma to genetics. Tumors account for about one third of all frontal lobe epilepsy cases. Low-grade tumors such as gangliogliomas, low-grade gliomas, and epidermoid tumors are most common, but many high-grade tumors were most likely once involved with seizures. Other lesions on the frontal lobe such as hamartomas and nodular heterotopias can cause frontal lobe symptoms as well. Birth defects such as vascular malformation are known to cause seizures, especially arteriovenous malformations and cavernous angiomas. Head trauma frequently causes damage to the frontal lobe and can cause seizures directly or indirectly through gliosis. Seizures originating directly from head trauma usually occur within a few months, but occasionally they can take years to manifest. On occasion encephalitis can cause frontal lobe seizures but it is most often associated with temporal lobe affliction. The main genetic cause of frontal lobe epilepsy is an autosomal dominant disease called Autosomal Dominant Nocturnal Frontal Lobe Epilepsy, which involves mutations in 2 nicotinic acetylcholine receptor genes. A genetic mutation on chromosome 22 has also been associated with another genetic form of the disorder.

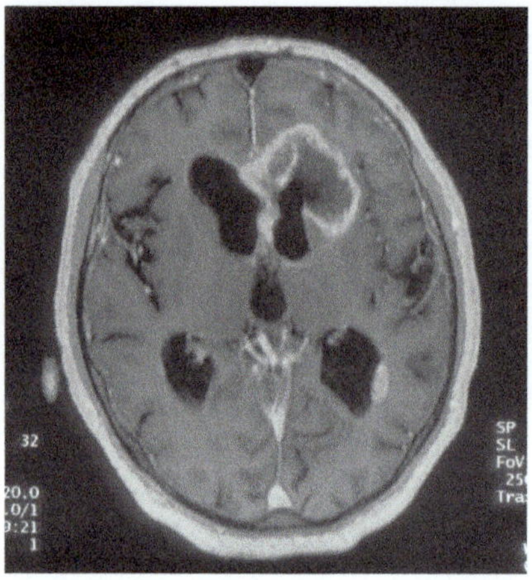

An MRI image of a brain with an invasive, multilocular tumor in the left Frontal lobe of the brain.

Mechanism

Due to the difference in brain processing and function as well as various surface anatomy landmarks, the frontal lobes have traditionally been divided into two major areas known as the precentral cortex and prefrontal cortex.

Precentral Cortex

The precentral cortex is an area of the frontal cortex that is located directly anterior to the central sulcus and includes both the primary motor cortex and the supplementary motor area. Inputs that project to both of these areas arise from a variety of locations in the brain that integrate sensory stimuli including the primary motor cortex, the thalamus and corticospinal projections. These two areas along with several other main functional areas control both the preparation of motor movement as well as the execution of movements. These main functional areas are crucial to the development of the motor related symptoms associated with frontal lobe epilepsy focally when seizures are located within these defined areas. The major functional areas include:

- Primary motor cortex
    - Contains large neurons that project axons down to the spinal cord where they synapse onto alpha motor neurons. These neurons are involved in the planning of motor movements and the refining of motor movements based on sensory inputs that are received from the cerebellum.

- Supplementary motor area
  - Area anterior to the primary motor cortex that is involved in planning complex motor movements and coordinating movements along both hands. The main inputs for this area are received from the thalamus.
- Frontal eye field
  - The frontal eye field is a posterior part of the middle frontal gyrus and is involved in the control of saccadic, contralateral and conjugate eye movement. This area receives its main inputs from both the occipital cortex and dorsal thalamus.
- Broca's area
  - Controls the motor movements of both the tongue and larynx that enables speech formation. This area receives direct inputs from the primary motor area as well as Wernicke's area located in the temporal lobe.

Prefrontal Cortex

The prefrontal cortex, the most anterior region of the brain, comprises several key areas that are particularly important for higher mental functions that control various aspects of human personality including anticipation and planning, initiative/judgement, memory and the control of decision making. Damage or lesions to this region of the brain can result in major changes in personality. A classic example is Phineas Gage, who exhibited a change in behavior after one or both frontal lobes were destroyed by a large iron bar accidentally driven through his head (though Gage, despite conventional presentations of his case, did not exhibit the aggression, antiosocial behavior, or loss of impulse control sometimes reported in patients with similar injuries).

There are two main regions of the prefrontal cortex that each control various aspects of behavior and personality:

- Dorsolateral prefrontal cortex
  - This area is associated with the impairment of the cognitive abilities that control and regulate behavior and long term memory formation (especially relating to procedural sequence memory) when either brain damage or a lesion is present.
- Orbitofrontal cortex
  - The orbitofrontal cortex has similar functions as the dorsolateral prefrontal cortex but is thought to be mainly responsible for the ability to make choices and determine right from wrong.

Social Effects and Quality of Life

Epilepsy has a substantial impact on the quality of life of the individuals that are afflicted with it. Physicians and researchers are coming to understand that the impact on the quality of life of the patient is as important as the effects of the seizures. Quality of life questionnaires and other assessment tools have been created to help quantify quality of life for individual patients. They consider such factors as physical health (including numbers and severity of seizures, medication side effects etc.), mental health, social relationships, lifestyle, role activities and life fulfillment. A Center for Disease Control study reported that seizure sufferers were more likely to have lower education levels, higher unemployment, higher levels of pain, hypersomnia/insomnia, increased psychological distress and social isolation/connection issues. Some of the issues which impact quality of life for people with epilepsy are: ability to drive and travel, the ability to date, marry and have children, the ability to have a job and independence, the ability to have an education and learn, and the ability to have good health and mental functioning. Future research is needed to find ways of not only controlling frontal lobe seizures, but of also addressing the specific quality-of-life issues that plague those with frontal lobe epilepsy.

Driving and transportation restrictions

- Driving and travel restrictions are one of the greatest limitations that epileptic patients experience. Laws restricting driving privileges vary greatly in the United States as well as across the world. In the United States, 28 states require a patient to be seizure free for fixed periods of time ranging from 3–12 months. However, research done by Johns Hopkins University showed that there was no difference in seizure-related fatal crash rates in states with 3-month restrictions versus states with 6-12 month seizure-free restrictions. In 23 states, the restrictions and seizure free periods vary depending on the type of epilepsy and the individual case and in 13 states physicians were responsible for determining whether their patients should be allowed to drive. In 6 of those 13 states physicians could be held legally liable for their decisions regarding their epileptic patients' driving capabilities. In many states, patients can also be legally liable for accidents, injury, damage and death caused by seizure related accidents.
- One of the major arguments in favor of restricting the licensing of epileptic drivers is the concern for public safety. However, the Johns Hopkins study showed that in a particular 2 year timeframe only 0.2% of fatal crashes occurred as a result of seizures. Alcohol related crash fatalities caused 156 times more driver deaths than seizure related crashes and young drivers between the ages of 16 and 24 were 123 times more likely to die in a fatal crash caused by their inexperience than an epileptic driver was to die in a crash that resulted from a seizure.
- Frontal lobe epileptic seizures unlike other epileptic seizures create symptoms that are as dangerous as loss of consciousness and much more difficult to discern from other problems such as drug and alcohol abuse, psychiatric disorders

and disobedience. Jerking movements/lack of motor control, pedaling, pelvic thrusting, lapses in cognitive functioning and other hallmark symptoms of frontal lobe epileptic seizures all create dangerous behavior behind the wheel. Studies have not been done to date to determine the differential risk posed by drivers with frontal lobe epilepsy relative to the general epileptic population.

Hormones and pregnancy issues

- Hormonal changes and pregnancy can shift seizure activity and the use of antiepileptic drugs can alter the efficacy of hormones as well as cause congenital malformations in fetuses. Seizure control in pregnant women is very important to the welfare of both the developing fetus and the mother. Hormonal shifts at puberty, with birth control and at menopause can also cause changes in the frequency and severity of seizures and must be closely monitored. Increased seizure activity is reported by 50% of women during the course of the pregnancy due to changing levels of hormones, fluids, salts and absorption and elimination of medications.

Employment

- A report by the Epilepsy Foundation noted that the unemployment rate amongst people with epilepsy is 25% and in patients whose seizures are poorly controlled the rate jumps to 50%. Even though people with epilepsy are protected under The Americans with Disabilities Act, employment discrimination and high rates of unemployment due to employer attitudes still exist. A study in the UK showed that 16% of employers surveyed felt there were no jobs in their company suitable for people with epilepsy and that 21% felt that employing an epileptic would be a "major issue". Fifty percent of the employers said they had a high concern regarding employing people with epilepsy with most citing safety concerns/workplace accidents as their major issue. Patients with frontal lobe epilepsy may be particularly prone to being discriminated against in employment and subject to higher rates of termination due to the unusual motor symptoms, speech, vocal outbursts and cognitive/judgment symptoms displayed during frontal lobe seizures. Frontal lobe seizures also tend to come on suddenly and progress rapidly making it difficult for an employer to control the exposure of the seizure to others.

Education, learning and cognitive function

- Patients with frontal lobe epilepsy will likely also experience issues with learning and education. Many factors contribute to these issues including the impact of anticonvulsant medications. Anticonvulsant medications cause patients to feel "foggy" and sluggish. Drugs such as Topiramate cause problems such as mental blunting, word retrieval difficulties and irritability. Phenobarbital, Primidone and Vigabatrin can cause depression and suicidal tendencies. Stress and lack of sleep during exam periods can trigger seizures and many school sports teams restrict or ban people with epilepsy from sports for safety and liability reasons. Frontal lobe epilepsy sufferers also exhibit dysfunctional cognitive skills and memory issues which can make learning challenging. Research has shown that frontal lobe epilepsy has a greater negative impact than other forms of epilepsy on cognitive functioning. People with frontal lobe epilepsy show decreased cognitive capabilities in the following areas: humor appreciation, recognition of emotional expressions, response selection/initiation and inhibition, hyperactivity, conscientiousness, obsession, addictive behavior, motor coordination and planning, attention span, performance speed, continuous performance without intrusion and interference errors, copying and recall, concept formation, anticipatory behavior, memory span, working memory, executive planning, visuo-spatial organization, mental flexibility, conceptual shift, problem solving, programming of complex motor sequences, impulse control, judgment and forecasting of consequences.

Physical health and risk of other conditions

- Patients with epilepsy face a greater risk of accidents, injury and other medical conditions than the general population. A European study showed that people with epilepsy were at greater risk for accidental injuries related to seizures such as concussions, abrasions and wounds and reported more hospitalizations and medical action than the general population. Other studies have shown that people with epilepsy are at a greater risk of seizure related drowning, suffocation, broken bones and burns and more likely to die in a fatal automobile crash.
- Epilepsy Ontario reports that people with epilepsy are also more likely to have other conditions than the general population such as: 30% of autistic children have epilepsy, 33% of cerebral palsy patients have epilepsy, 15-20% of fragile X syndrome patients have epilepsy, 50% of children with learning disabilities will have some form of epilepsy, 3-10% of patients with Lennox-Gastaut syndrome will have epilepsy, 80% of children with Rett syndrome will have epilepsy and 80% of patients with Tuberous Sclerosis will have epilepsy.

Mental and emotional health

- Epileptic patients are more prone to suffer psychological and social dysfunction than individuals that do not have epilepsy. They report higher levels of anxiety and stress due to social isolation, discrimination, the unpredictability of their seizures and people's reactions to them as well as fear of injury, death and brain damage from their seizures. Anticonvulsants can also result in lower functioning, depression, sluggishness and suicidal thoughts. Approximately 20% of people with epilepsy are depressed and the rate of suicide amongst people with epilepsy is 5 times the rate in the general population.
- People with frontal lobe epilepsy experience more significant social effects be-

cause the manifested symptoms are more unusual. Symptoms such as screaming, bicycling limbs, pelvic thrusting, inhibition control and other outbursts can be particularly embarrassing and isolating for the patient.

Treatments

There are several different ways to treat frontal lobe epileptic seizures, however, the most common form of treatment is through the use of anticonvulsant medications that help to prevent seizures from occurring. In some cases, however, when medications are ineffective, a neurologist may choose to operate on the patient in order to remove the focal area of the brain in which the seizures are occurring. Other treatments that can be administered to aid in reducing the occurrence of seizures include the implementation of a specific, regimented diet and/or the implantation of a vagus nerve stimulator.

Medications

Anticonvulsants are the most successful medication in reducing and preventing seizures from reoccurring. The goal of these medications in being able to reduce the reoccurrence of seizures is to be able to limit the amount of rapid and extensive firing of neurons so that a focal region of neurons cannot become over-activated thereby initiating a seizure. Although anticonvulsants are able to reduce the amount of seizures that occur in the brain, no medication has been discovered to date that is able to prevent the development of epilepsy following a head injury. There are a wide range of anticonvulsants that have both different modes of action and different abilities in preventing certain types of seizures. Some of the anticonvulsants that are prescribed to patients today include: Carbamazepine (Tegretol), Phenytoin (Dilantin Kapseals), Gabapentin (Neurontin), Levetiracetam (Keppra), Lamotrigine (Lamictal), Topiramate (Topamax), Tiagabine (Gabitril), Zonisamide (Zonegran) and Pregabalin (Lyrica).

Note on Medications

Lorazepam and clonazepam are front line treatment for severe convulsions, belonging to the benzodiazepine class of medications.

Surgical Treatment

When both the amount and severity of seizures becomes uncontrollable and seizures remain resistant to the various anticonvulsants, a patient most likely will be considered for epilepsy surgery such as a frontal lobectomy. This procedure involves the removal of focal regions of the frontal lobes that have been identified as being problematic for the patient. It has been found that around 30% to 50% of patients that undergo a frontal lobectomy will forever be free from seizures that cause a loss of consciousness or cause abnormal movements.

If on the other hand, the seizures occur in an area that is too vital to remove (such as areas that control motor, sensory or language functions), then the surgeon will perform a procedure known as a multiple subpial transection. This procedure involves making a series of cuts that surround the focal region where the seizures have originated. By making cuts surrounding the focal region, the surgeon is able to isolate that specific section of the brain and prevent electrical impulses from being able to travel horizontally to other areas of the brain.

The last surgical procedure that can be done to help prevent the reoccurrence of seizures in the frontal lobes is to implant a stimulator on the vagus nerve. This device is a self-activating device that is inserted directly under the skin and can be controlled directly by the patient. When a patient is feeling the onset of an aura, he/she can activate the stimulator which in turn will provide stimulation to the left vagus nerve (the left vagus nerve is used because the right nerve plays a role in cardiac function). Although little is understood about the exact mechanism for vagal nerve stimulation, it has been proven to be a successful treatment that can often terminate seizures before they begin.

Diet

The use of a regimented diet is an approach that has been found to help control seizures in children with severe, medically intractable frontal lobe epilepsy. Although the use of dieting to prevent seizures from occurring is a lost treatment that has been replaced by the use of new types of anticonvulsants, it is still recommended to patients to this day. A ketogenic diet is a high-fat, low-carbohydrate based diet that patients are typically asked to follow in conjunction with their anticonvulsant medications. This diet was designed in order to mimic many of the effects that starvation has on the metabolic functioning of the body. By limiting the amount of carbohydrates and increasing the amount of exogenous fats available to the metabolism, the body will create an excess of water-soluble compounds known as ketone bodies. Although the mechanism of action is still unknown, it is believed that these excessive amounts of ketone bodies become the brain's main source of energy and in turn are able to suppress the frequency of seizure occurrence.

Epidemiology

Epilepsy is a relatively common disorder, affecting between 0.5-1% of the population, and frontal lobe epilepsy accounts for about 1-2% of all epilepsies. The most common subdivision of epilepsy is symptomatic partial epilepsy, which causes simple partial seizures, and can be further divided into temporal and frontal lobe epilepsy. Although the exact number of cases of frontal lobe epilepsy is not currently known, it is known that FLE is the less common type of partial epilepsy, accounting for 20-30% of operative procedures involving intractable epilepsy. The disorder also has no gender or age bias, affecting males and females of all ages. In a recent study, the mean subject age with frontal lobe epilepsy was 28.5 years old, and the average age of epilepsy onset for left frontal epilepsy was 9.3 years old whereas for right frontal epilepsy it was 11.1 years old.

Nocturnal Epilepsy

Nocturnal epilepsy is a seizure disorder in which seizures occur only while sleeping. Several common forms of epilepsy, including frontal lobe epilepsy, can manifest in a nocturnal state.

Epilepsy can be nocturnal if the form of epilepsy triggers seizures only while one is asleep, or if one normally has seizures that occur at that time. In the latter example, if the subject stays awake at a time when he is normally sleeping, the subject may have the seizure while awake. Noting this, it is important for the subject to maintain a proper sleeping cycle. Diverting from proper sleep patterns can trigger more frequent epileptic symptoms in people who are diagnosed with nocturnal epilepsy and, as mentioned before, even while awake.

Diagnosis

The condition may be difficult to diagnose. The subject may be unaware they have a seizure disorder. To others, the involuntary movements made during sleep may appear no different from those typical of normal sleep.People who have nocturnal seizures may notice unusual conditions upon awakening in the morning, such as a headache, having wet the bed, having bitten the tongue, a bone or joint injury, muscle strains or weakness, fatigue, or lightheadedness. Others may notice unusual mental behaviors consistent with the aftermath of a seizure. Objects near the bed may have been knocked to the floor, or the subject may be surprised to find themselves on the floor.

There are many risks associated with nocturnal seizures including concussion, suffocation and sudden unexpected death(SUDEP). It is often also very difficult to know how long the seizure has been going.

Type

A person who suffers from epilepsy regardless of whether it is nocturnal or not, can be categorized into two different types of epilepsy either being generalized, or partial. A generalized epilepsy syndrome is associated with an overall hyperactivity in the brain, where electrical discharges occur all over the brain at once; this syndrome often has a genetic basis. While generalized epilepsy occurs all over the brain, partial epilepsy consists of a regional or localized hyperactivity, which means that the seizures occur conversely in one part of the brain or several parts at once.

Treatment

Like other forms of epilepsy, nocturnal epilepsy can be treated with anti-convulsants. Despite the effectiveness of anti-convulsants in people who suffer from nocturnal epilepsy, the drugs are shown to disrupt a person's sleeping structure. This may cause concern in people who suffer specifically from nocturnal epilepsy because undisrupted sleep is important for these people, as it lowers the likeliness of epileptic symptoms to arise.

One particular study by V. Bradley and D. O'Neill analysed the different forms of epilepsy, including nocturnal epilepsy and its relationship with sleep. They found that some patients only experienced epileptic symptoms while they are asleep (nocturnal epilepsy), and that maintaining good sleep helped in reducing epileptic symptoms. Another study determined that anti-convulsant medications can minimize epilepsy not just in people who are awake, but also in people who are asleep. However, some of these anti-convulsant medications did also have adverse effects on subjects' sleeping structures, which can exacerbate epileptic symptoms in people who suffer from nocturnal epilepsy.

To minimize epileptic seizures in these people, it is important to find an anti-convulsant medication that does not disrupt a person's sleeping structure. The anti-convulsant medications that were tested to meet this criteria are: phenobarbital, phenytoin, carbamazepine, valproate, ethosuximide, felbamate, gabapentin, lamotrigine, topiramate, vigabatrin, tiagabine, levetiracetam, zonisamide, and oxcarbazepine. Oxcarbazepine is shown to have the least amount of adverse effects on sleep. Another study shows that it enhances slow wave-sleep and sleep continuity in patients with epilepsy.

Photosensitive Epilepsy

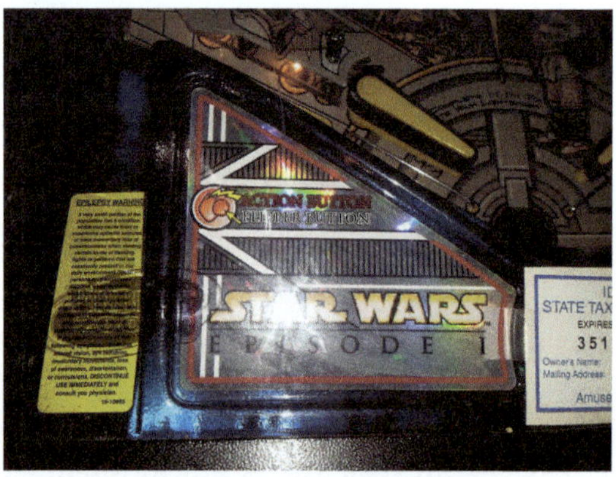

Epilepsy warning label on a pinball machine with video components.

Photosensitive epilepsy (PSE) is a form of epilepsy in which seizures are triggered by visual stimuli that form patterns in time or space, such as flashing lights, bold, regular patterns, or regular moving patterns.

Signs and Symptoms

People with PSE experience epileptiform seizures upon exposure to certain visual stimuli. The exact nature of the stimulus or stimuli that triggers the seizures varies from one patient to another, as does the nature and severity of the resulting seizures (ranging from brief absence seizures to full tonic–clonic seizures). Many PSE patients experience an "aura" or feel odd sensations before the seizure occurs, and this can serve as a warning to a patient to move away from the trigger stimulus.

The visual trigger for a seizure is generally cyclic, forming a regular pattern in time or space. Flashing lights or rapidly changing or alternating images (as in clubs, around emergency vehicles, in action movies or television programs, etc.) are examples of patterns in time that can trigger seizures, and these are the most common triggers. Static spatial patterns such as stripes and squares may trigger seizures as well, even if they do not move. In some cases, the trigger must be both spatially and temporally cyclic, such as a certain moving pattern of bars.

Also note: Some people may also find overhead fans spinning to be of the same nature.

Several characteristics are common in the trigger stimuli of many PSE patients. The patterns are usually high in luminance contrast (bright flashes of light alternating with darkness, or white bars against a black background). Contrasts in colour alone (without changes in luminance) are rarely triggers for PSE. Some patients are more affected by patterns of certain colours than by patterns of other colours. The exact spacing of a pattern in time or space is important and varies from one individual to another: a patient may readily experience seizures when exposed to lights that flash seven times per second, but may be unaffected by lights that flash twice per second or twenty times per second. Stimuli that fill the entire visual field are more likely to cause seizures than those that appear in only a portion of the visual field. Stimuli perceived with both eyes are usually much more likely to cause seizures than stimuli seen with one eye only (which is why covering one eye may allow patients to avoid seizures when presented with visual challenges). Some patients are more sensitive with their eyes closed; others are more sensitive with their eyes open.

Sensitivity is increased by alcohol consumption, sleep deprivation, illness, and other forms of stress.

Television

Television has traditionally been the most common source of seizures in PSE. For people with PSE, it is especially hazardous to view television in a dark room, at close range, or when the television is out of adjustment and is showing a rapidly flickering image (as when the horizontal hold is incorrectly adjusted). Modern digital television sets that cannot be maladjusted in this way and refresh the image on the screen at very high speed present less of a risk than older television sets.

Some people with PSE, especially children, may exhibit an uncontrollable fascination with television images that trigger seizures, to such an extent that it may be necessary to physically keep them away from television sets. Some people (particularly those with cognitive impairments, although most people with PSE have no such impairments) self-induce seizures by waving their fingers in front of their eyes in front of bright light or by other means.

Some UK television broadcasters and studios now screen content through the "Harding FPA Test", an objective standard of assessment of potential to trigger seizures in the susceptible population.

In some cases, specific television programs featuring certain types of visual stimuli have provoked seizures in a small minority of television viewers, including some viewers with no prior history of seizures of any kind. The "Dennō Senshi Porygon" episode of *Pokémon* is the most frequently cited example; when the program was broadcast in Japan, its strong flickering scenes produced seizures in a surprising number of viewers, even though the proportion of viewers affected was extremely low.

Fluorescent Lighting

When functioning correctly, mains-powered fluorescent lighting has a flicker rate sufficiently high (twice the mains frequency, typically 100 Hz or 120 Hz) to reduce the occurrence of problems. However, a faulty fluorescent lamp can flicker at a much lower rate and trigger seizures. Newer high-efficiency compact fluorescent lamps (CFL) with electronic ballast circuits operate at much higher frequencies (10–20 kHz) not normally perceivable by the human eye, though defective lights can still cause problems.

The Job Accommodation Network lists reduction or elimination of fluorescent lighting as an appropriate accommodation for many conditions including epilepsy. The Canadian Department of Labour states that the newer lights are problematic for fewer people.

Video Games and Pinball Machines

The first case of epileptiform seizures related to a video game was reported in 1981. Since then, "many cases of seizures triggered by video games were reported, not only in photosensitive, but also in nonphotosensitive children and adolescents with epilepsy.....Specific preventive measures concerning the physical characteristics of images included in commercially available video games (flash rate, choice of colours, patterns, and contrast) can lead in the future to a clear decrease of this problem." Risks can be reduced through measures such as keeping a safe distance away from the screen (at least 2 meters).

While computer displays in general present very little risk of producing seizures in PSE patients (much less risk than that presented by television sets), video games with rapidly changing images or highly regular patterns can produce seizures, and video games have increased in importance as triggers as they have become more common. Some people with no prior history of PSE may first experience a seizure while playing a video game. Often the sensitivity is very specific, *e.g.*, it may be a specific scene in a specific game that causes seizures, and not any other scenes. Despite this, there are questions on the dangers of this, and calls for testing all video games for causing PSE. Laws requiring PSE warnings be displayed on packages and/or stores have been proposed and legal firms are keeping an eye on developments. The Star Wars: Episode I – The Phantom Menace pinball machine, which had video components, included an epilepsy warning label, as did Attack From Mars.

Web Design

As with video games, rapidly changing images or highly regular patterns such as flashing banner ads or irregular fonts can trigger seizures in people with photosensitive epilepsy. Two sets of guidelines exist to help web designers produce content that is safe for people with photosensitive epilepsy:

- The World Wide Web Consortium - Web Content Accessibility Guidelines (WCAG) Version 2.0, produced in 2008, specifies that content should not flash more than 3 times in any 1 second period. However it does allow flashing above this rate if the flashing is below the "general and red flashing thresholds". (Basically, it is OK to flash more than 3 times in a 1-second period if the flashing is small enough or low contrast enough.)
- In the United States, websites provided by federal agencies are governed by section 508 of the Rehabilitation Act. The Act says that pages shall be designed to avoid causing the screen to flicker with a frequency greater than 2 Hz and less than 55 Hz. The 508 regulations are currently being updated and are expected to use the same criteria as WCAG 2.0 when finished.
- A free tool for evaluating Web Content for flashing called the Photosensitive Epilepsy Analysis Tool (PEAT) is available from the Trace R&D Center at the University of Maryland.

Diagnosis

Diagnosis may be made by noting the correlation between exposure to specific visual stimuli and seizure activity. More precise investigation can be carried out by combining an EEG with a device producing *Intermittent Photic Stimulation* (IPS). The IPS device produces specific types of stimuli that can be controlled and adjusted with precision. The testing physician adjusts the IPS device and looks for characteristic anomalies in the EEG, such as photoparoxysmal response (PPR), that are consistent with PSE and/or may herald the onset of seizure activity. The testing is halted before a seizure actually occurs.

Sometimes diagnostic indicators consistent with PSE can be found through provocative testing with IPS, and yet no seizures may ever occur in real-life situations. Many people will show PSE-like abnormalities in brain activity with sufficiently aggressive stimulation, but they never experience seizures and are not considered to have PSE.

Treatment and Prognosis

No cure is available for PSE, although the sensitivity of some patients may diminish over time. Medical treatment is available to reduce sensitivity, with sodium valproate being commonly prescribed. Patients can also learn to avoid situations in which they might be exposed to stimuli that trigger seizures and/or take steps to diminish their sensitivity (as by covering one eye) if they are unavoidably exposed. These actions together can reduce the risk of seizures to almost zero for many PSE patients.

Some PSE patients have trigger stimuli that are so specific that they are never likely to encounter them in real life. Their PSE may only be discovered by accident in an unusual situation or during examination for other complaints.

Society and Culture

The effect of stroboscopic lighting became apparent to the general public when it first became popular in discotheques during the 1960s. Many authorities responded by regulating the permissible frequency ranges of flashing lights in public places.

Photosensitive epilepsy was again brought to public attention in December 1997 when the *Pokémon* episode "Dennō Senshi Porygon" ("Cyber Soldier Porygon") was broadcast in Japan, showing a sequence of flickering images that triggered seizures simultaneously in hundreds of susceptible viewers (although 12,000 children reported symptoms which may be attributable to mass hysteria).

In March 1997, the 25th episode of an anime series called *YAT Anshin! Uchū Ryokō* caused a similar incident, when a reported four children were taken to hospitals by ambulances after viewing a scene with red and white flashing colours.

In March 2008, the Anonymous group of hackers was claimed to be behind an attack on a forum for epilepsy sufferers. The Anonymous hackers in turn blamed the Church of Scientology for the attacks, saying they were falsified to hurt Anonymous' image. The attacks first consisted of GIF images flashing at high speeds that were hidden in discussion threads with innocuous-sounding titles. Later attacks redirected web browsers to a page with "a more complex image designed to trigger seizures in both photosensitive and pattern-sensitive epileptics". The technology website Wired News considered it to be "possibly the first computer attack to inflict physical harm on the victims".

An animated segment of a film promoting the 2012 London Olympics was blamed for triggering seizures in people with photosensitive epilepsy. The charity Epilepsy Action received telephone calls from people who had seizures after watching the film on television and online. In response, the London 2012 Olympic Committee removed the offending segment from its website.

Post-traumatic Epilepsy

Post-traumatic epilepsy (PTE) is a form of epilepsy that results from brain damage caused by physical trauma to the brain (traumatic brain injury, abbreviated TBI). A person with PTE suffers repeated post-traumatic seizures (PTS, seizures that result from TBI) more than a week after the initial injury. PTE is estimated to constitute 5% of all cases of epilepsy and over 20% of cases of symptomatic epilepsy (in which seizures are caused by an identifiable organic brain condition).

It is not known how to predict who will develop epilepsy after TBI and who will not. However, the likelihood that a person will develop PTE is influenced by the severity and type of injury; for example penetrating injuries and those that involve bleeding within the brain confer a higher risk. The onset of PTE can occur within a short time of the physical trauma that causes it, or months or years after. People with head trauma may remain at a higher risk for seizures than the general population even decades after the injury. PTE may be caused by several biochemical processes that occur in the brain after trauma, including overexcitation of brain cells and damage to brain tissues by free radicals.

Diagnostic measures include electroencephalography (EEG) and brain imaging techniques such as magnetic resonance imaging, but these are not totally reliable. Antiepileptic drugs do not prevent the development of PTE after head injury, but may be used to treat the condition if it does occur. When medication does not work to control the seizures, surgery may be needed. Modern surgical techniques for PTE have their roots in the 19th century, but trepanation (cutting a hole in the skull) may have been used for the condition in ancient cultures.

Classification

Seizures may occur after traumatic brain injury; these are known as post-traumatic seizures (PTS). However, not everyone who has post-traumatic seizures will continue to have post-traumatic epilepsy, because the latter is a chronic condition. However, the terms PTS and PTE are used interchangeably in medical literature. Seizures due to post-traumatic epilepsy are differentiated from non-epileptic post-traumatic seizures based on their cause and timing after the trauma. A person with PTE suffers late seizures, those occurring more than a week after the initial trauma. Late seizures are considered to be unprovoked, while early seizures (those occurring within a week of trauma) are thought to result from direct effects of the injury. A provoked seizure is one that results from an exceptional, nonrecurring cause such as the immediate effects of trauma rather than a defect in the brain; it is not an indication of epilepsy. Thus for a diagnosis of PTE, seizures must be unprovoked.

Disagreement exists about whether to define PTE as the occurrence of one or more late, unprovoked seizures, or whether the condition should only be diagnosed in people with two or more. Medical sources usually consider PTE to be present if even one unprovoked seizure occurs, but more recently it has become accepted to restrict the definition of all types of epilepsy to include only conditions in which more than one occur. Requiring more than one seizure for a diagnosis of PTE is more in line with the modern definition of epilepsy, but it eliminates people for whom seizures are controlled by medication after the first seizure.

As with other forms of epilepsy, seizure types in PTE may be partial (affecting only part of one hemisphere of the brain) or generalized (affecting both hemispheres and associated with loss of consciousness). In about a third of cases, people with PTE have partial seizures; these may be simple or complex. In simple partial seizures, level of consciousness is not altered, while in complex partial seizures consciousness is impaired. When generalized seizures occur, they may start out as partial seizures and then spread to become generalized.

Causes

It is not clear why some patients get PTE while others with very similar injuries do not. However, possible risk factors have been identified, including severity and type of injury, presence of early seizures, and genetic factors.

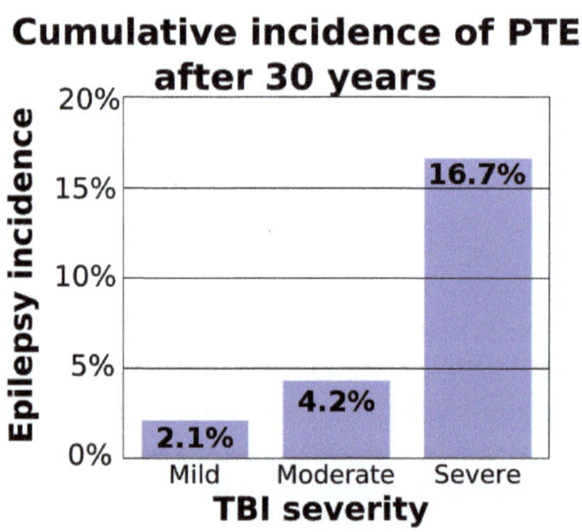

Cumulative incidence after 30 years of PTE in head injured individuals

Genetics

Genetics may play a role in the risk that a person will develop PTE; people with the ApoE-ε4 allele may be at higher risk for PTE. The haptoglobin Hp2-2 allele may be another genetic risk factor, possibly because it binds hemoglobin poorly and thus allows more iron to escape and damage tissues. However, most studies have found that having family members with epilepsy does not significantly increase the risk of PTS, suggesting that genetics are not a strong risk factor.

Severity of Trauma

The more severe the brain trauma is, the more likely a person is to suffer late PTE. Evidence suggests that mild head injuries do not confer an increased risk of developing PTE, while more severe types do. In simple mild TBI, the risk for PTE is about 1.5 times that of the uninjured population. By some estimates, as many as half of sufferers of severe brain trauma experience PTE; other estimates place the risk at 5% for all TBI patients and 15–20% for severe TBI. One study found that the 30-year risk of developing PTE was 2.1% for mild TBI, 4.2% for moderate, and 16.7% for severe injuries, as shown in the chart.

Nature of Trauma

The nature of the head trauma also influences the risk of PTE. People who suffer depressed skull fractures, penetrating head trauma, early PTS, and intracerebral and subdural haematomas due to the TBI are especially likely to suffer PTE, which occurs in more than 30% of people with any one of these findings. About 50% of patients with penetrating head trauma develop PTE, and missile injuries and loss of brain volume are associated with an especially high likelihood of developing the condition. Injuries that occur in military settings carry higher-than-usual risk for PTE, probably because they more commonly involve penetrating brain injury and brain damage over a more widespread area. Intracranial hematomas, in which blood accumulates inside the skull, are one of the most important risk factors for PTE. Subdural hematoma confers a higher risk of PTE than does epidural hematoma, possibly because it causes more damage to brain tissue. Repeated intracranial surgery confers a high risk for late PTE, possibly because people who need more surgery are more likely to have factors associated with worse brain trauma such as large hematomas or cerebral swelling. In addition, the chances of developing PTE differ by the location of the brain lesion: brain contusion that occurs on in one or the other of the frontal lobes has been found to carry a 20% PTE risk, while a contusion in one of the parietal lobes carries a 19% risk and one in a temporal lobe carries a 16% chance. When contusions occur in both hemispheres, the risk is 26% for the frontal lobes, 66% for the parietal, and 31% for the temporal.

Post-traumatic Seizures

The risk that a person will develop PTE is heightened but not 100% if PTS occur. Because many of the risk factors for both PTE and early PTS are the same, it is unknown whether the occurrence of PTS is a risk factor in and of itself. However, even independent of other common risk factors, early PTS have been found to increase the risk of PTE to over 25% in most studies. A person who has one late seizure is at even greater risk for having another than one who has early PTS; epilepsy occurs in 80% of people who have a late seizure. Status epilepticus, a continuous seizure or multiple seizures in rapid succession, is especially strongly correlated with the development of PTE; status seizures occur in 6% of all TBIs but are associated with PTE 42% of the time, and quickly halting a status seizure reduces chances of PTE development.

Pathophysiology

For unknown reasons, trauma can cause changes in the brain that lead to epilepsy. There are a number of proposed mechanisms by which TBI causes PTE, more than one of which may be present in a given person. In the period between a brain injury and onset of epilepsy, brain cells may form new synapses and axons, undergo apoptosis or necrosis, and experience altered gene expression. In addition, damage to particularly vulnerable areas of the cortex such as the hippocampus may give rise to PTE.

Blood that gathers in the brain after an injury may damage brain tissue and thereby cause epilepsy. Products that result from the breakdown of hemoglobin from blood may be toxic to brain tissue. The "iron hypothesis" holds that PTE is due to damage by oxygen free radicals, the formation of which is catalyzed by iron from blood. Animal experiments using rats have shown that epileptic seizures can be produced by injecting iron into the brain. Iron catalyzes the formation of hydroxyl radicals by the Haber-Weiss reaction; such free radicals damage brain cells by peroxidizing lipids in their membranes. The iron from blood also reduces the activity of an enzyme called nitric oxide synthase, another factor thought to contribute to PTE.

After TBI, abnormalities exist in the release of neurotransmitters, chemicals used by brain cells to communicate with each other; these abnormalities may play a role in the development of PTE. TBI may lead to the excessive release of glutamate and other excitatory neurotransmitters (those that stimulate brain cells and increase the likelihood that they will fire). This excessive glutamate release can lead to excitotoxicity, damage to brain cells through overactivation of the biochemical receptors that bind and respond to excitatory neurotransmitters. Overactivation of glutamate receptors damages neurons; for example it leads to the formation of free radicals. Excitotoxicity is a possible factor in the development of PTE; it may lead to the formation of a chronic epileptogenic focus. An epileptic focus is the part of the brain from which epileptic discharges originate.

In addition to chemical changes in cells, structural changes that lead to epilepsy may occur in the brain. Seizures that occur shortly after TBI can reorganize neural networks and cause seizures to occur repeatedly and spontaneously later on. The kindling hypothesis suggests that new neural connections are formed in the brain and cause an increase in excitability. The word *kindling* is a metaphor: the way the brain's response to stimuli increases over repeated exposures is similar to the way small burning twigs can produce a large fire. This reorganization of neural networks may make them more excitable. Neurons that are in a hyperexcitable state due to trauma may create an epileptic focus in the brain that leads to seizures. In addition, an increase in neurons' excitability may accompany loss of inhibitory neurons that normally serve to reduce the likelihood that other neurons will fire; these changes may also produce PTE.

Diagnosis

To be diagnosed with PTE, a person must have a history of head trauma and no history of seizures prior to the injury. Witnessing a seizure is the most effective way to diagnose PTE. Electroencephalography (EEG) is a tool used to diagnose a seizure disorder, but a large portion of people with PTE may not have the abnormal "epileptiform" EEG findings indicative of epilepsy. In one study, about a fifth of people who had normal EEGs three months after an injury later developed PTE. However, while EEG is not useful for predicting who will develop PTE, it can be useful to localize the epileptic focus, to determine severity, and to predict whether a person will suffer more seizures if they stop taking antiepileptic medications.

Magnetic resonance imaging (MRI) is performed in people with PTE, and CT scanning can be used to detect brain lesions if MRI is unavailable. However, it is frequently not possible to detect the epileptic focus using neuroimaging.

For a diagnosis of PTE, seizures must not be attributable to another obvious cause. Seizures that occur after head injury are not necessarily due to epilepsy or even to the head trauma. Like anyone else, TBI survivors may suffer seizures due to factors including imbalances of fluid or electrolytes, epilepsy from other causes, hypoxia (insufficient oxygen), and ischemia (insufficient blood flow to the brain). Withdrawal from alcohol is another potential cause of seizures. Thus these factors must be ruled out as causes of seizures in people with head injury before a diagnosis of PTE can be made.

Prevention

Prevention of PTE involves preventing brain trauma in general; protective measures include bicycle helmets and child safety seats. No specific treatment exists to prevent the development of epilepsy after TBI occurs. In the past, antiepileptic drugs were used with the intent of preventing the development of PTE. However, while antiepileptic drugs can prevent early PTS, clinical studies have failed to show that prophylactic use of antiepileptic drugs prevents the development of PTE. Why antiepileptic drugs in clinical trials have failed to stop PTE from developing is not clear, but several explanations have been offered. The drugs may simply not be capable of preventing epilepsy, or the drug trials may have been set up in a way that did not allow a benefit of the drugs to be found (e.g. drugs may have been given too late or in inadequate doses). Animal studies have similarly failed to show much protective effect of the most commonly used seizure medications in PTE trials, such as phenytoin and carbamazepine. Antiepileptic drugs are recommended to prevent late seizures only for people in whom PTE has already been diagnosed, not as a preventative measure. On the basis of the aforementioned studies, no treatment is widely accepted to prevent the development of epilepsy. However, it has been proposed that a narrow window of about one hour after TBI may exist during which administration of antiepileptics could prevent epileptogenesis (the development of epilepsy).

Corticosteroids have also been investigated for the prevention of PTE, but clinical trials revealed that the drugs did not reduce late PTS and were actually linked to an increase in the number of early PTS.

Treatment

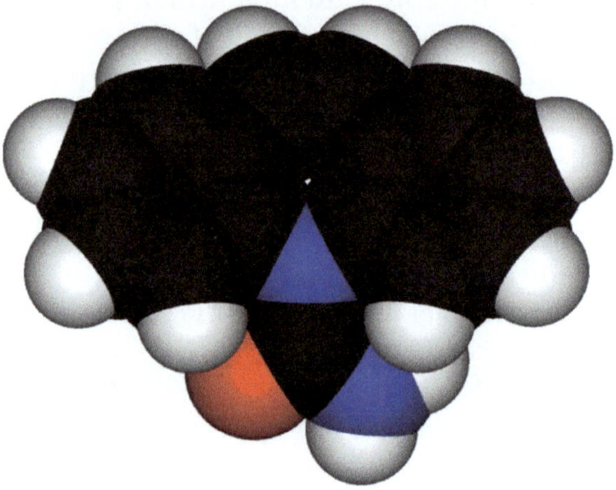

Carbamazepine, commonly used to treat PTE

Antiepileptic drugs may be given to prevent further seizures; these drugs completely eliminate seizures for about 35% of people with PTE. However, antiepileptics only prevent seizures while they are being taken; they do not reduce the occurrence once the patient stops taking the drugs. Medication may be stopped after seizures have been controlled for two years. PTE is commonly difficult to treat with drug therapy, and antiepileptic drugs may be associated with side effects. The antiepileptics carbamazepine and valproate are the most common drugs used to treat PTE; phenytoin may also be used but may increase risk of cognitive side effects such as impaired thinking. Other drugs commonly used to treat PTE include clonazepam, phenobarbitol, primidone, gabapentin, and ethosuximide. Among antiepileptic drugs tested for seizure prevention after TBI (phenytoin, sodium valproate, carbamazepine, phenobarbital), no evidence from randomized controlled trials has shown superiority of one over another.

People whose PTE does not respond to medication may undergo surgery to remove the epileptogenic focus, the part of the brain that is causing the seizures. However surgery for PTE may be more difficult than it is for epilepsy due to other causes, and is less likely to be helpful in PTE than in other forms of epilepsy. It can be particularly difficult in PTE to localize the epileptic focus, in part because TBI may affect diffuse areas of the brain. Difficulty locating the seizure focus is seen as a deterrent to surgery. However, for people with sclerosis in the mesial temporal lobe (in the inner aspect of the temporal lobe), who comprise about one third of people with intractable PTE, surgery is likely to have good outcome. When there are multiple epileptic foci or the focus cannot be localized, and drug therapy is not effective, vagus nerve stimulation is another option for treating PTE.

People with PTE have follow-up visits, in which health care providers monitor neurological and neuropsychological function and assess the efficacy and side effects of medications. As with sufferers of other types of epilepsy, PTE sufferers are advised to exercise caution when performing activities for which seizures could be particularly risky, such as rock climbing.

Prognosis

The prognosis for epilepsy due to trauma is worse than that for epilepsy of undetermined cause. People with PTE are thought to have shorter life expectancies than people with brain injury who do not suffer from seizures. Compared to people with similar structural brain injuries but without PTE, people with PTE take longer to recover from the injury, have more cognitive and motor problems, and perform worse at everyday tasks. This finding may suggest that PTE is an indicator of a more severe brain injury, rather than a complication that itself worsens outcome. PTE has also been found to be associated with worse social and functional outcomes but not to worsen patients' rehabilitation or ability to return to work. However, people with PTE may have trouble finding employment if they admit to having seizures, especially if their work involves operating heavy machinery.

The period of time between an injury and development of epilepsy varies, and it is not uncommon for an injury to be followed by a latent period with no recurrent seizures. The longer a person goes without developing seizures, the lower the chances are that epilepsy will develop. At least 80–90% of people with PTE have their first seizure within two years of the TBI. People with no seizures within three years of the injury have only a 5% chance of developing epilepsy. However, one study found that head trauma survivors are at an increased risk for PTE as many as 10 years after moderate TBI and over 20 years after severe TBI. Since head trauma is fairly common and epilepsy can occur late after the injury, it can be difficult to determine whether a case of epilepsy resulted from head trauma in the past or whether the trauma was incidental.

The question of how long a person with PTE remains at higher risk for seizures than the general population is controversial. About half of PTE cases go into remission, but cases that occur later may have a smaller chance of doing so.

Epidemiology

Studies have found that the incidence of PTE ranges between 1.9 and more than 30% of TBI sufferers, varying by severity of injury and by the amount of time after TBI for which the studies followed subjects.

Brain trauma is one of the strongest predisposing factors for epilepsy development, and is an especially important factor in young adults. Young adults, who are at the highest risk for head injury, also have the highest rate of PTE, which is the largest cause of new-onset epilepsy cases in young people. Children have a lower risk for developing epilepsy; 10% of children with severe TBI and 16–20% of similarly injured adults develop PTE. Being older than 65 is also a predictive factor in the development of epilepsy after brain trauma. One study found PTE to be more common in male TBI survivors than in females.

History

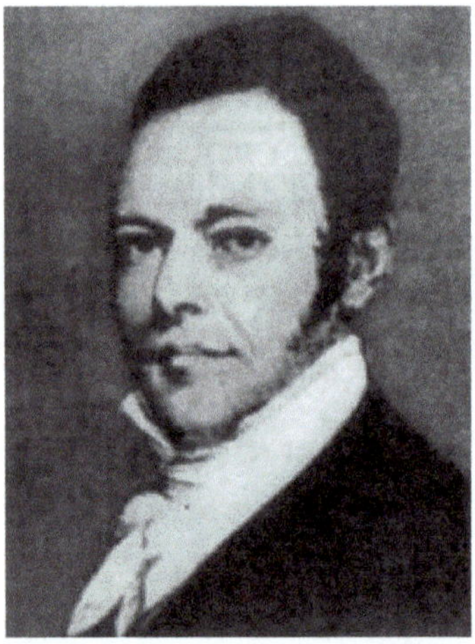

Benjamin Winslow Dudley performed trepanation for PTE before antisepsis was available.

Records of PTE exist from as early as 3000 BC. Trepanation, in which a hole is cut in the skull, may have been used to treat PTE in ancient cultures. In the early 19th century, the surgeons Baron Larrey and WC Wells each reported having performed the operation for PTE. The French-educated American surgeon Benjamin Winslow Dudley (1785–1870) performed six trepanations for PTE between the years of 1819 and 1832 in Kentucky and had good results despite the unavailability of antisepsis. The surgery involved opening the skull at the site of injury, debriding injured tissue, and sometimes draining blood or fluid from under the dura mater. Dudley's work was the largest series of its kind that had been done up to that point, and it encouraged other surgeons to use trepanation for post-traumatic seizures. His reports on the operations came before it was accepted that surgery to relieve excess pressure within the skull was effective in treating epilepsy, but it helped set the stage for trepanation for PTE to become common practice. The procedure became more accepted in the late 19th century once antisepsis was available and cerebral localization was a familiar concept. However, in 1890, the prominent German physician Ernest von Bergmann criticized the procedure; he questioned its efficacy (except in particular circumstances) and suggested that operations had been declared successful too soon after the procedures to know whether they would confer a long-term benefit. The late 19th century saw the advent of *intracranial* surgery, operating on brain lesions believed to be causing seizures, a step beyond *cranial* surgery which involved just the skull and meninges. By 1893, at least 42 intracranial operations had been performed for PTE in the US, with limited success.

Surgery was the standard treatment for PTE until the years following World War II, when the condition received more attention as soldiers who had survived head trauma developed it. The increased need for drugs to treat PTE led to trials with antiepileptics; these early trials suggested that the drugs could prevent epileptogenesis (the development of epilepsy). It was still thought that antiepileptic drugs could prevent epileptogeneis in the 1970s; in 1973, 60% of physicians surveyed used them to prevent PTE. However, the clinical trials which had supported a protective effect of antiepileptics were uncontrolled; in later, controlled trials the drugs failed to demonstrate an antiepileptogenic effect. Studies did show that antiepileptics prevented seizures occurring within a week after injury, and in 1995 the task force of the Brain Trauma Foundation published a recommendation suggesting their use to protect against seizures early after trauma. However, recommendations were published against the prophylactic use of antiepileptic drugs more than a week after injury by the Brain Injury Special Interest group of the American Academy of Physical Medicine and Rehabilitation in 1998 and by the American Association of Neurological Surgeons in 2000.

Myoclonic Epilepsy

Myoclonic epilepsy refers to a family of epilepsies that present with myoclonus. When myoclonic jerks are occasionally associated with abnormal brain wave activity, it can be categorized as myoclonic seizure. If the abnormal brain wave activity is persistent and results from ongoing seizures, then a diagnosis of myoclonic epilepsy may be considered.

Classification

There are two syndromes and several related disorders.

Juvenile

Juvenile myoclonic epilepsy is responsible for 7% of cases of epilepsy. Seizures usually begin around puberty and usually have a genetic basis. Seizures can be stimulus-selective, with flashing lights being one of the most common triggers.

Progressive

Progressive myoclonus epilepsy is a disease associated with myoclonus, epileptic seizures, and other problems with walking or speaking. These symptoms often worsen over time and can be fatal.

MERRF syndrome is also known as myoclonic epilepsy with ragged-red fibers. This rare inherited disorder affects muscles cells. Features of MERRF, along with myoclonus epilepsy seizures, include ataxia, peripheral neuropathy, and dementia.

Lafora disease is also known as Lafora progressive myoclonus epilepsy, which is an autosomal recessive inherited disorder involving recurrent seizures and degradation of mental capabilities. Lafora disease usually occurs in late childhood and usually leads to death around 10 years after first signs of the disease.

Unverricht-Lundborg disease is an autosomal recessive inherited disorder seen in individuals as young as six years. It is associated with possible loss of consciousness, rigidity, ataxia, dysarthria, declination of mental functioning, and involuntary shaking.

Neuronal ceroid lipofuscinosis is a group of diseases that cause blindness, loss of mental abilities, and loss of movement. All diseases in this group are lysosomal-storage disorders that also lead to death roughly ten years after onset of the disease.

Related Disorders

Lennox–Gastaut syndrome is often associated with intellectual deficits as well as a lack of response to anti-epileptic drugs. It usually begins in the first years of life.

Reticular reflex myoclonus is a generalized form of epilepsy originating from the brain stem. Jerks associated with the disorder can affect all muscles on the body or be selective in certain areas. Jerks can be triggered by voluntary movement or be stimulus-selective.

Signs and Symptoms

Myoclonus can be described as brief jerks of the body; it can involve any part of the body, but it is mostly seen in limbs or facial muscles. The jerks are usually involuntary and can lead to falls. EEG is used to read brain wave activity. Spike activity produced from the brain is usually correlated with brief jerks seen on EMG or excessive muscle artifact. They usually occur without detectable loss of consciousness and may be generalized, regional or focal on the EEG tracing. Myclonus jerks can be epileptic or not epileptic. Epileptic myoclonus is an elementary electroclinical manifestation of epilepsy involving descending neurons, whose spatial (spread) or temporal (self-sustained repetition) amplification can trigger overt epileptic activity.

Differential Diagnosis

Myoclonic jerks that are not epileptic may be due to a nervous system disorder or other metabolic abnormalities that may arise in renal (e.g. hyperuraemia) and liver failure (e.g. high ammonia states).

References

- Kobayashi M.; Buckmaster P. S (2003). "Reduced inhibition of dentate granule cells in a model of temporal lobe epilepsy". Journal of Neuroscience. 23 (6): 2440–2452. PMID 12657704
- Janz, D.; Christian, W. (1994). "Impulsive petit mal". In Malafosse, Alain. Idiopathic Generalized Epilepsies: Clinical, Experimental and Genetic Aspects. pp. 229–51. ISBN 978-0-86196-436-9
- Perez-Reyes E (2006). "Molecular characterization of T-type calcium channels". Cell Calcium. 40 (2): 89–96. PMID 16759699. doi:10.1016/j.ceca.2006.04.012
- Buckmaster P, et al. (2002). "Axon sprouting in a model of temporal lobe epilepsy creates a predominantly excitatory feedback circuit". Journal of Neuroscience. 22 (15): 6650–6658. PMID 12151544
- Blum D (1999). "Total Impact of Epilepsy: Biological, Psychological, Social and Economic Aspects". Barrow Quarterly. Retrieved 2009-12-01
- Shinnar S, et al. (2008). "Phenomenology of prolonged febrile seizures: results of the FEBSTAT study". Neurology. 71 (3): 170–176. PMID 18525033. doi:10.1212/01.wnl.0000310774.01185.97
- Nadler J. V.; et al. (1985). "Evidence of functional mossy fiber sprouting in hippocampal formation of kainic acid-treated rats". Journal of Neuroscience. 5 (4): 1016–1022. PMID 3981241
- De Lanerolle N. C. and Noebels J. L. (ed.) Jasper's basic mechanisms of the epilepsies: histopathology of human epilepsy. Oxford University Press 2012 chapter 30 ISBN 978-0-19-974654-5
- "Gamma Knife Radiosurgery for Epilepsy". University of Virginia School of Medicine. 2007-10-11. Archived from the original on 2008-10-10. Retrieved 2009-12-03
- Babb T. L.; et al. (1991). "Synaptic reorganization by mossy fibers in human epileptic fascia dentata". Neuroscience. 42 (2): 351–363. PMID 1716744. doi:10.1016/0306-4522(91)90380-7
- Ng, B. Y. (2002). "Psychiatric aspects of self-induced epileptic seizures". The Australian and New Zealand Journal of Psychiatry. 36 (4): 534–543. PMID 12169155. doi:10.1046/j.1440-1614.2002.01050.x
- Waterman K, Wada J (1991). "Frontal lobe epilepsy". In Gram L, Dam M. Comprehensive epileptology. New York: Raven Press. pp. 197–213. ISBN 0-88167-646-2
- Niedermeyer, Ernst (1992). "Epileptic Syndromes: A Remarkable Contribution of EEG to Epileptology". American Journal of EEG Technology (32): 10–12
- "Policy Reports/Study Group/Broadcasting Bureau". Ministry of Internal Affairs and Communications. April 1998. Archived from the original on 2008-10-23. Retrieved 2008-11-02

3

Various Epilepsy Syndromes

Epileptic syndromes are analyzed to understand the causes of epilepsy. They also help to identify the suitable medication to be given to treat epilepsy. Epilepsy syndromes are easily detected in children. The topics discussed in the chapter are of great importance to broaden the existing knowledge on epilepsy.

Benign Infantile Epilepsy

Benign infantile epilepsy (BIE), also known as benign infantile seizures (BIS), is an epilepsy syndrome of which several forms have been described. The International League Against Epilepsy (ILAE) classify two main forms of the syndrome (familial and nonfamilial) though several other forms have been described in the academic literature. Affected children, who have no other health or developmental problems, develop seizures during infancy. These seizures have focal origin within the brain but may then spread to become generalised seizures. The seizures may occur several times a day, often grouped in clusters over one to three days followed by a gap of one to three months. Treatment with anticonvulsant drugs is not necessary but they are often prescribed and are effective at controlling the seizures. This form of epilepsy resolves after one or two years, and appears to be completely benign. The EEG of these children, between seizures, is normal. The brain appears normal on MRI scan.

The familial and nonfamilial forms have overlapping features and the presence of a family history of infantile seizures may be the only distinguishing criterion. The nonfamiliar form has a larger range of the onset of seizures: from three to twenty months with most occurring between five and six months. There is no difference between the sexes. With benign familial infantile epilepsy, the seizures onset from four to eight months of age.

Some cases of nonfamilial benign infantile seizures occur during a case of mild gastroenteritis. Called *benign infantile seizures associated with mild gastroenteritis* (BIS with MG), the seizures only occur during this illness and no not recur. Infection with rotavirus is the most common cause.

Although children with benign infantile epilepsy typically have a normal EEG between seizures, some infants have been found to have a characteristic abnormal EEG during sleep. Called *benign infantile focal epilepsy with midline spikes and waves during sleep*, these infants have few seizures and there may often be a family history.

Benign Familial Infantile Epilepsy

Benign familial infantile epilepsy (BFIE), also known as benign familial infantile seizures (BFIS) or benign familial infantile convulsions (BFIC) is an epilepsy syndrome. Affected children, who have no other health or developmental problems, develop seizures during infancy. These seizures have focal origin within the brain but may then spread to become generalised seizures. The seizures may occur several times a day, often grouped in clusters over one to three days followed by a gap of one to three months. Treatment with anticonvulsant drugs is not necessary but they are often prescribed and are effective at controlling the seizures. This form of epilepsy resolves after one or two years, and appears to be completely benign. The EEG of these children, between seizures, is normal. The brain appears normal on MRI scan.

A family history of epilepsy in infancy distinguishes this syndrome from the non-familial classification, though the latter may be simply sporadic cases of the same genetic mutations. The condition is inherited with an autosomal dominant transmission. There are several genes responsible for this syndrome, on chromosomes 2, 16 and 19. It is generally described as idiopathic, meaning that no other neurological condition is associated with it or causes it. However, there are some forms that are linked to neurological conditions. One variant known as infantile convulsions and choreoathetosis (ICCA) forms an association between BFIE and paroxysmal kinesigenic choreoathetosis and has been linked to the PRRT2 gene on chromosome 16. An association with some forms of familial hemiplegic migraine (FHM) has also been found. Benign familial infantile epilepsy is not genetically related to benign familial neonatal epilepsy (BFNE), which occurs in neonates. However, a variation with seizure onset between two days and seven months called *benign familial neonatal–infantile seizures* (BFNIS) has been described, which is due to a mutation in the SCN2A gene.

Catamenial Epilepsy

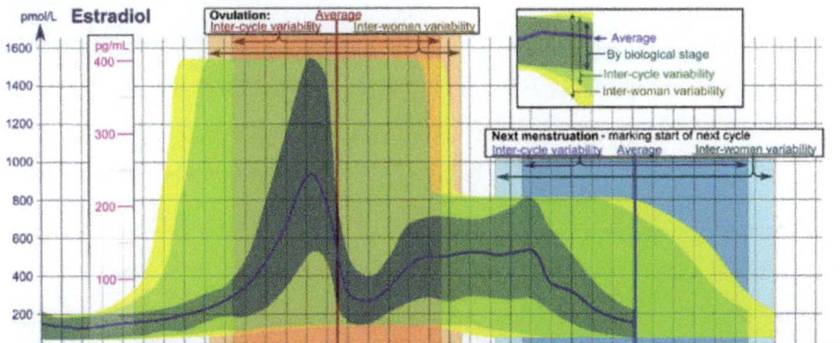

Estradiol levels during the menstrual cycle.

Epilepsy is a chronic neurological condition characterized by recurrent seizures. Catamenial epilepsy is a subset of epilepsy, which includes women whose seizures are exacerbated by their menstrual cycle. Women with catamenial epilepsy are unusually sensitive to endogenous hormonal changes. This seizure exacerbation has a statistically significant positive correlation to serum estradiol/estrogen levels and ratios.

Since at least the Greek times, there has been documented study of women with epilepsy and its correlation to the menstrual cycle. These patterns can easily be seen by charting out menses against seizure occurrence and type.

Pathophysiology

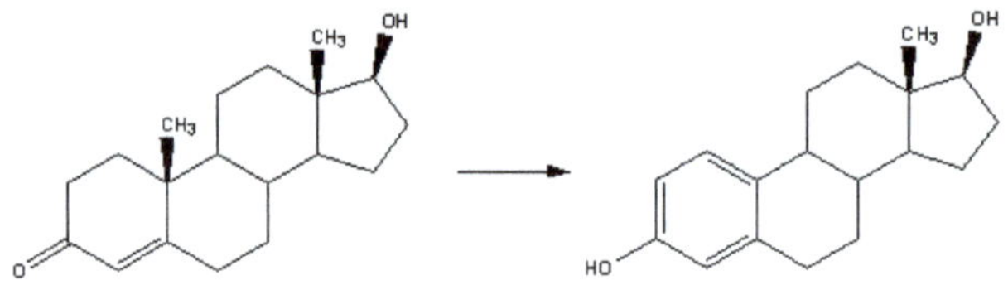

Conversion of testosterone to estradiol

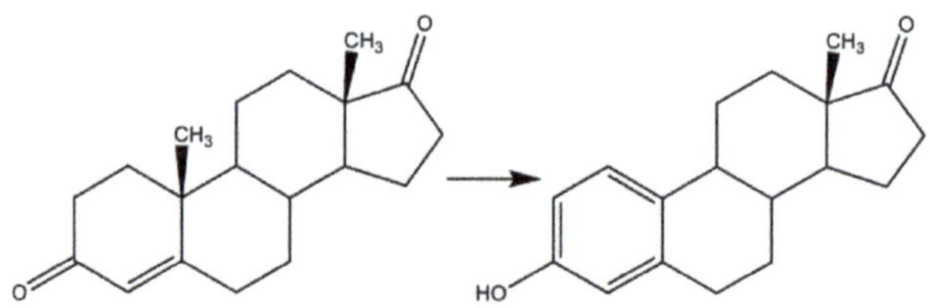

Aromatase converts androstenedione to estrone

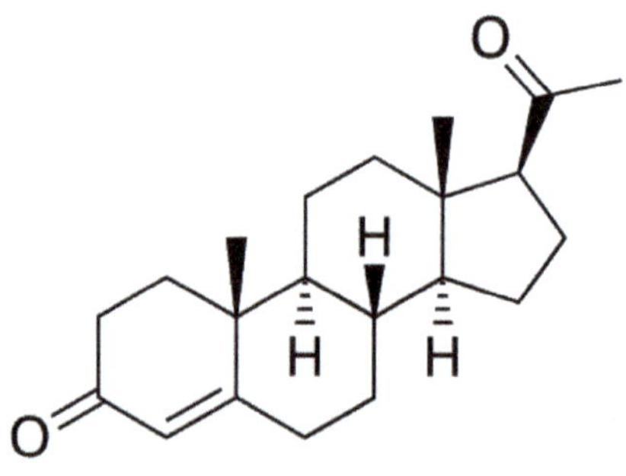

Progesterone

Our understanding of the major gonadal hormones, estrogen, progesterone, and testosterone, has significantly increased in the last century. These hormones are synthesized in various locations in the body, including the ovaries, adrenal gland, liver, subcutaneous fat, and brain. There is considerable research showing that these steroidal hormones take part in an important role in the pathophysiology of epilepsy. Broadly defined, estrogen and its many forms are thought to be "proconvulsant," whereas progesterone is thought to be "anticonvulsant" by virtue of its conversion to the neurosteroid allopregnanolone.

Estrogen (Estradiol, Estrone, Estriol)

Estrogen can be found in the female body in various forms, all of which affect women with catamenial epilepsy. Estrone (E1), estradiol (E2), and estriol (E3) are the three principal circulating estrogens in the body. These three forms influence neuronal excitability, but very little is known about their inter-hormone interactions, the relative concentrations and ratios of E1/E2/E3 and how that may influence the seizure frequency behavior in women with epilepsy. In normally menstruating women, serum estradiol levels are typically present by day 10 of the menstrual cycle, and persist until ovulation.

- *Estrone*'s main source is adipose tissue (subcutaneous fat), where it is formed by aromatization of androstenedione. Estrone is the major estrogen after menopause, and this hormone may be very influential in seizure control of the catamenial woman if she is severely overweight or obese.
- *Estradiol* represents the most prolific estrogen ligand receptor in the female body, particularly in non-pregnant females, and is a more effective activator of estrogen receptor function than estrone or estriol. Estradiol directly increases NMDA mediated receptors of glutamate activity at the neuronal membrane. Through this mechanism hippocampal pyramidal neurons CA1 are excited, and a repetitive firing response is induced. Dendritic spine density on CA1 hippocampal pyramidal cells is dependent upon estradiol levels, showing a direct correlation during normal fluctuations during the menstrual cycle. Estradiol has been shown to apply its effects on dendritic spine density of hippocampal cells by using a mechanism that requires activation of NMDA receptors. Furthermore, Herzog postulates that, "estradiol may thus further increase excitatory input to the CA1 neurons." Through many animal models, as well as human-use of estrogen-based hormone replacement therapy, estrogens have been seen to increase the excitability of neurons, leading to a decreased seizure threshold. In female adult rat experimental trials, the limbic seizure threshold fluctuates inversely to estradiol levels during the estrous cycle.
- *Estriol* is known to inhibit GABA and to promote kindling and epileptiform discharges. Estriol is only produced in significant quantities during pregnancy via placental aromatization of fetal androgen, however it can also be synthesized in smaller quantities (non-pregnancy) in the liver by hydroxylation of estrone.

Progesterone

Similar to estrogen, progesterone receptors bind several molecules other than only progesterone. Progestogens are group of natural non-synthetic hormones, including progesterone, which binds to progesterone receptors. Other than progesterone, progestogens have several neuroactive metabolites, most notably allopregnanolone. Progesterone has been shown to lower the number of estrogen receptors, and thus act as an antagonist to estrogen actions. In trials, both progesterone and allopregnanolone administration have shown a neuroprotective effect on hippocampal neurons in seizure models induced by kainic acid.

Classification

The proper classification for catamenial epilepsy has been debatable for several decades. Researchers have defined catamenial epilepsy from the broadest definition of a "greater than" approach indicating an increase in seizure frequency or severity during any specific phase of the menstrual cycle, to a "sixfold increase" in average daily seizure frequency during specific times in the cycle. In recent years, Herzog's 1997 proposal of an admittedly arbitrary "twofold" increase has generally been accepted: Perimenstrual (C1), Periovulatory (C2), and Luteal (C3). These three classifications are based upon serum estradiol:progesterone ratio, and a 24- to 34-day menstrual cycle in which menses begins on day 1, and ovulation occurs 14 days prior to menstruation. By this measure, approximately one third of women with epilepsy would be classified under the designation of catamenial epilepsy.

Perimenstrual "C1"

Perimenstrual classification (in normal cycles, days -3 to 3 of menstruation) is associated with a twofold or greater increase in average daily seizure occurrence during the menstrual phase (M) compared to the follicular (F) and luteal (L) phases. The menstrual phase is characterized by drastic decreases in progesterone and estrogen levels. The estradiol:progesterone ratio is highest during the days before menstruation (C1) and ovulation (C2). Perimenstrual seizure exacerbation has been recognized as the withdrawal of the protective effects of progesterone. In a 2009 study, it was found that patients with C1 pattern of catamenial epilepsy had overall lower progesterone levels than healthy controls during the M phase.

Periovulatory "C2"

Periovulatory classification (in normal cycles, days 10 to -13) is associated with a twofold or greater increase in average daily seizure occurrence during the O phase compared to the F and L phases. The ovulatory phase is characterized by a surge of estrogen before ovulation, while an associated progesterone surge does not occur until ovulation actually occurs. This estrogen effect, without a corresponding progesterone surge of protection, intensifies seizure events.

Luteal "C3"

Luteal classification (abnormal or inadequate luteal phase cycles, days 10 to 3) is associated with a twofold or greater increase in average daily seizure occurrence during the O, L and M phases. Anovulatory females do not typically have a midcycle surge of progesterone, but still experience a surge in estrogen. These women have abnormally low progesterone levels during the O, L and M, regardless of whether ovulation occurs. In study by El-Khayat et al., it was found that patients with C3 pattern of catamenial epilepsy had overall lower progesterone levels than healthy controls during the L phase of the menstrual cycle.

Menopause

During menopause, there are drastic changes in the production of gonadal hormones. Most of the reproductive hormones, including the estrogens, progesterone and testosterone, diminish initially (perimenopause), becoming irregular, often showing wide and unpredictable fluctuations. As menopause progresses, there is cessation of estrogen production by the ovaries. Rosciszewska was one of the first researchers to report an increased risk of seizures during perimenopause, but found a marked decreased risk of seizures during menopause if there was a catamenial relationship. This difference may be associated with the radical fluctuations of estradiol and progesterone during the perimenopausal period than what is experienced during the menopausal period and menstrual cycles of reproductive years. Recall that estrone is the predominant estrogen present during menopause (from subcutaneous fat), and little is known about the effect of estrone specifically on epilepsy. Women with epilepsy who do not follow a catamenial pattern may have an unpredictable increase or decrease in seizure activity in perimenopause and menopause, but women with catamenial epilepsy typically follow a more predictable pattern.

Hormone Replacement Therapy

The use of hormone replacement therapy (HRT), to lessen the effects of menopause, has shown severe negative effects on the seizure patterns of women with catamenial epilepsy. During perimenopause, women with catamenial epilepsy generally experience an increase in seizure frequency, and HRT use does not change this likelihood. However HRT use after perimenopause has been significantly associated with an increase in seizure frequency and severity. Women progressing through peri- and post-menopause using HRT may be in greater need of anticonvulsant medication monitoring to maintain or reduce seizure occurrence. These same results have not been seen in laboratory counterparts. Adult female rats that have been ovariectomized, a parallel state to menopause, show increased seizure frequency overall. There are, however, several factors that could explain this difference, including ovariectomized rats do not have the analogous brain hormones milieu as menopausal women. Several studies following HRT use in women with catamenial epilepsy have demonstrated more influencable data than animal models, in this case.

Treatment

Several treatment methods have been determined exclusively for women with catamenial epilepsy. A great majority of these therapies include progestagens (naturally occurring) or progestins (synthetic progestagen). Drug interactions are an important factor when using progesterone therapy, as many antiseizure medications augment hepatic metabolism of gonadal steroids, and increase serum protein binding to hormones. There are many unfortunate side effects frequently seen in progesterone therapy usage, including vaginal dryness, dyspareunia, osteoporosis, and cardiovascular disease.

- *Cyclic progesterone therapy* supplements the patient with natural progesterone during the luteal phase when progesterone is normally low, and gradually reduces the supplementation premenstrually.
- *Suppressive progestin therapy* intends to suppress the menstrual cycle entirely by using injectable progestins or gonadotropin-releasing hormones (GnRH). GnRH basically mimics an ovary-free environment in the female, which is characteristic of the lack of menstrual cycle during menopause.

Progressive Myoclonus Epilepsy

Progressive myoclonus epilepsy (PME) is a rare epilepsy syndrome caused by a variety of genetic disorders. The syndrome includes myoclonic seizures and tonic-clonic seizures together with progressive neurological decline.

Signs and Symptoms

Myoclonic seizures involve brief involuntary muscle twitching, and may become frequent enough to be disabling. Tonic-clonic seizures have two phases: the tonic phase may last a few seconds and involves the muscles tensing, and may lead to the person falling down; the clonic phase involves a convulsion of rapidly alternating muscle tensing and relaxing. Neurological dysfunction includes difficulty coordinating muscle movements (ataxia) and a decline in cognitive ability (dementia).

Differential Diagnosis

In the early stages, it can be difficult to distinguish progressive myoclonic epilepsy from benign idiopathic generalised epilepsies, such as juvenile myoclonic epilepsy. With PME, the initial effectiveness of anticonvulsant treatment diminishes as seizures become more frequent and neurological decline progresses. However, these can also be signs of anticonvulsant intoxication. The myoclonus in PME is usually severe and is the prominent seizure type.

Specific Disorders

Six specific disorders comprise the most common causes of progressive myoclonic epilepsy: Unverricht-Lundborg disease (Baltic myclonus); myoclonus epilepsy and ragged red fibres (MERRF syndrome); Lafora disease; neuronal ceroid lipofuscinoses; and type I sialidosis. Less common causes include dentatorubropallidoluysian atrophy (DRPLA); the noninfantile neuronopathic form of Gaucher disease; and atypical inclusion body disease. PME has also been reported in Niemann-Pick disease type C.

Unverricht-lundborg Disease

This disease manifests between six and sixteen years and is most prevalent in Scandinavia and the Baltic countries. Myoclonus gradually becomes worse and less susceptible to medication. Cognitive decline is slow and sometimes mild. Patients typically do not live beyond middle-age, but there are exceptions. Phenytoin, an old and commonly used anticonvulsant, is known to seriously exacerbate the condition. It has autosomal recessive inheritance, and is caused by a mutation in the cystatin B (EPM1) gene on chromosome 21q22.3, which was discovered in 1996.

It has been described as the least severe type of PME.

Myoclonus Epilepsy and Ragged Red Fibres (MERRF Syndrome)

Onset of this disease may be at any time and the severity and progression are varied. Tonic-clonic seizures and dementia are less apparent than with other forms of PME. The cause is a mitochondrial DNA mutation, so most familial cases are transmitted from the mother. A skeletal muscle biopsy will show ragged red fibres, hence the name.

Lafora Body Disease

This disease typically begins between six and nineteen years after apparently normal development and generally results in death within ten years. It is characterised by the presence of Lafora bodies (polyglucosan inclusions) in neurons and other body tissue. The generalized seizures are usually well controlled by anticonvulsants, but the myoclonus soon proves refractory to treatment. Within a couple of years, a wheelchair is required for locomotion and within five to ten years, the person is confined to bed and is often tube fed. Valproic acid and zonisamide are first choice anticonvulsants, and the ketogenic diet may be helpful. An autosomal-recessive genetic defect is responsible, which has been tracked down to two genes. The EPM2A gene on chromosome 6q24 was discovered in 1998 and encodes for the protein laforin. It is responsible for 80% of cases. The EPM2B gene on chromosome 6p22.3 was discovered in 2003 and encodes for the protein malin. There may be a third gene of unknown locus.

Neuronal Ceroid Lipofuscinoses

There are various forms of these disorders, each with their own genetic cause and geographical variation, which lead to accumulation of lipopigments (lipofuscin) in the body's tissues and are inherited in an autosomal-recessive fashion. Onset and symptoms vary with the particular form, but death usually occurs within five to fifteen years.

Type I Sialidosis

This is an autosomal recessive disorder in which the body is deficient in α-neuraminidase.

Epidemiology

PME accounts for less than 1% of epilepsy cases at specialist centres. The incidence and prevalence of PME is unknown, but there are considerable geography and ethnic variations amongst the specific genetic disorders. One cause, Unverricht Lundborg Disease, has an incidence of at least 1:20,000 in Finland.

Rolandic Epilepsy

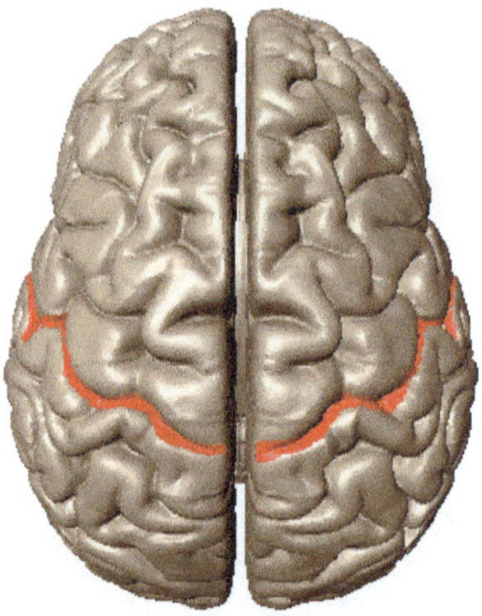

Central sulcus of the brain, superior view.

Benign Rolandic epilepsy or benign childhood epilepsy with centrotemporal spikes (BCECTS) is the most common epilepsy syndrome in childhood. Most children will outgrow the syndrome (it starts around the age of 3-13 with a peak around 8–9 years and stops around age 14-18), hence the label benign. The seizures, sometimes referred to as *sylvian seizures*, start around the central sulcus of the brain (also called the centrotemporal area, located around the Rolandic fissure, after Luigi Rolando).

Signs and Symptoms

The cardinal features of Rolandic epilepsy are infrequent, often single, focal seizures consisting of:

a. unilateral facial sensorimotor symptoms (30% of patients)

b. oropharyngolaryngeal manifestations (53% of patients)

c. speech arrest (40% of patients), and

d. hypersalivation (30% of patients)

Hemifacial sensorimotor seizures are often entirely localised in the lower lip or spread to the ipsilateral hand. Motor manifestations are sudden, continuous or bursts of clonic contractions, usually lasting from a few seconds to a minute. Ipsilateral tonic deviation of the mouth is also common. Hemifacial sensory symptoms consist of unilateral numbness mainly in the corner of the mouth. Hemifacial seizures are often associated with an inability to speak and hypersalivation: *The left side of my mouth felt numb and started jerking and pulling to the left, and I could not speak to say what was happening to me.* Negative myoclonus can be observed in some cases, as an interruption of tonic muscular activity

Oropharyngolaryngeal ictal manifestations are unilateral sensorimotor symptoms inside the mouth. Numbness, and more commonly paraesthesias (tingling, prickling, freezing), are usually diffuse on one side or, exceptionally, may be highly localised even to one tooth. Motor oropharyngolaryngeal symptoms produce strange sounds, such as death rattle, gargling, grunting and guttural sounds, and combinations: *In his sleep, he was making guttural noises, with his mouth pulled to the right, 'as if he was chewing his tongue'. We heard her making strange noises 'like roaring' and found her unresponsive, head raised from the pillow, eyes wide open, rivers of saliva coming out of her mouth, rigid.*

Arrest of speech is a form of anarthria. The child is unable to utter a single intelligible word and attempts to communicate with gestures. *My mouth opened and I could not speak. I wanted to say I cannot speak. At the same time, it was as if somebody was strangling me.*

Hypersalivation , a prominent autonomic manifestation, is often associated with hemifacial seizures, oro-pharyngo-laryngeal symptoms and speech arrest. Hypersalivation is not just frothing: *Suddenly my mouth is full of saliva, it runs out like a river and I cannot speak.*

Syncope-like epileptic seizures may occur, probably as a concurrent symptom of Panayiotopoulos syndrome: *She lies there, unconscious with no movements, no convulsions, like a wax work, no life.*

Consciousness and recollection are fully retained in more than half (58%) of Rolandic seizures. *I felt that air was forced into my mouth, I could not speak and I could not close my mouth. I could understand well everything said to me. Other times I feel that there is food in my mouth and there is also a lot of salivation. I cannot speak.* In the remainder (42%), consciousness becomes impaired during the ictal progress and in one third there is no recollection of ictal events.

Progression to hemiconvulsions or generalised tonic–clonic seizures occurs in around half of children and hemiconvulsions may be followed by postictal Todd's hemiparesis.

Duration and circadian distribution: Rolandic seizures are usually brief, lasting for 1–3 min. Three quarters of seizures occur during nonrapid eye movement sleep, mainly at sleep onset or just before awakening.

Status epilepticus: Although rare, focal motor status or hemiconvulsive status epilepticus is more likely to occur than secondarily generalised convulsive status epilepticus, which is exceptional. Opercular status epilepticus usually occurs in children with atypical evolution or may be induced by carbamazepine or lamotrigine. This state lasts for hours to months and consists of ongoing unilateral or bilateral contractions of the mouth, tongue or eyelids, positive or negative subtle perioral or other myoclonus, dysarthria, speech arrest, difficulties in swallowing, buccofacial apraxia and hypersalivation. These are often associated with continuous spikes and waves on an EEG during NREM sleep.

Other seizure types: Despite prominent hypersalivation, focal seizures with primarily autonomic manifestations (autonomic seizures) are not considered part of the core clinical syndrome of Rolandic epilepsy. However, some children may present with independent autonomic seizures or seizures with mixed Rolandic-autonomic manifestations including emesis as in Panayiotopoulos syndrome.

Atypical forms: Rolandic epilepsy may present with atypical manifestations such early age at onset, developmental delay or learning difficulties at inclusion, other seizure types, atypical EEG abnormalities.

These children usually have normal intelligence and development. Learning can remain unimpaired while a child is afflicted with Rolandic epilepsy.

Cause

Benign epilepsy with centrotemporal spikes is thought to be a genetic disorder. An autosomal dominant inheritance with age dependency and variable penetrance has been reported, although not all studies support this theory. Linkage studies have pointed to a possible susceptibility region on chromosome 15q14, in the vicinity of the alpha-7 subunit of the acetylcholine receptor. Most studies show a slight male predominance. Because of the benign course and age-specific occurrence, it is thought to represent a hereditary impairment of brain maturation.

An association with ELP4 has been identified.

Diagnosis

The diagnosis can be confirmed when the characteristic centrotemporal spikes are seen on electroencephalography (EEG). Typically, high-voltage spikes followed by slow waves are seen. Given the nocturnal activity, a sleep EEG can often be helpful. Technically, the label "benign" can only be confirmed if the child's development continues to be normal during follow-up. Neuroimaging, usually with an MRI scan, is only advised for cases with atypical presentation or atypical findings on clinical examination or EEG. The disorder should be differentiated from several other conditions, especially centrotemporal spikes without seizures, centrotemporal spikes with local brain pathology, central spikes in Rett syndrome and fragile X syndrome, malignant Rolandic epilepsy, temporal lobe epilepsy and Landau-Kleffner syndrome.

Treatment

Given the benign nature of the condition and the low seizure frequency, treatment is often unnecessary. If treatment is warranted or preferred by the child and his or her family, antiepileptic drugs can usually control the seizures easily. Carbamazepine is the most frequently used first-line drug, but many other antiepileptic drugs, including valproate, phenytoin, gabapentin, levetiracetam and sultiame have been found effective as well. Bedtime dosing is advised by some. Treatment can be short and drugs can almost certainly be discontinued after two years without seizures and with normal EEG findings, perhaps even earlier. Parental education about Rolandic epilepsy is the cornerstone of correct management. The traumatizing, sometimes long-lasting effect on parents is significant.

It is unclear if there are any benefits to clobazam over other seizure medications.

Prognosis

The prognosis for Rolandic seizures is invariably excellent, with probably less than 2% risk of developing absence seizures and less often GTCS in adult life. Remission usually occurs within 2–4 years from onset and before the age of 16 years. The total number of seizures is low, the majority of patients having fewer than 10 seizures; 10–20% have just a single seizure. About 10–20% may have frequent seizures, but these also remit with age. Children with Rolandic seizures may develop usually mild and reversible linguistic, cognitive and behavioural abnormalities during the active phase of the disease. These may be worse in children with onset of seizures before 8 years of age, high rate of occurrence and multifocal EEG spikes. The development, social adaptation and occupations of adults with a previous history of Rolandic seizures were found normal.

Epidemiology

The age of onset ranges from 1 to 14 years with 75% starting between 7–10 years. There is a 1.5 male predominance, prevalence is around 15% in children aged 1–15 years with non-febrile seizures and incidence is 10–20/100,000 of children aged 0–15 years.

Landau–Kleffner Syndrome

Landau–Kleffner syndrome (LKS)—also called infantile acquired aphasia, acquired epileptic aphasia or aphasia with convulsive disorder—is a rare childhood neurological syndrome.

It is named after William Landau and Frank Kleffner, who characterized it in 1957 with a diagnosis of six children.

Signs and Symptoms

It is characterized by the sudden or gradual development of aphasia (the inability to understand or express language) and an abnormal electroencephalogram (EEG). LKS affects the parts of the brain that control comprehension and speech (Broca's area and Wernicke's area). The disorder usually occurs in children between the ages of 3 and 7 years. There appears to be a slight male dominance in the diagnosis of the syndrome (ratio of 1.7:1, men to women).

Typically, children with LKS develop normally, but then lose their language skills. While many affected individuals have clinical seizures, some only have electrographic seizures, including electrographic status epilepticus of sleep (ESES). The first indication of the language problem is usually auditory verbal agnosia. This is demonstrated in patients in multiple ways including the inability to recognize familiar noises and the impairment of the ability to lateralize or localize sound. In addition, receptive language is often critically impaired, however in some patients, impairment in expressive language is the most profound. In a study of 77 cases of Landau–Kleffner syndrome, 6 were found to have this type of aphasia. Because this syndrome appears during such a critical period of language acquisition in a child's life, speech production may be affected just as severely as language comprehension. The onset of LKS is typically between 18 months and 13 years, the most predominant time of emergence being between 3 and 7 years.

Generally, earlier manifestation of the disease correlates with poorer language recovery, and with the appearance of night seizures that last for longer than 36 months. LKS has a wide range of symptom differences and lacks a uniformity in diagnostic criteria between cases, and many studies don't include follow-ups on the patients, so no other relationships between symptoms and recovery have been made known.

Language deterioration in patients typically occurs over a period of weeks or months. However, acute onset of the condition has also been reported as well as episodic aphasia.

Seizures, especially during the night, are a heavily weighted indicator of LKS. The prevalence of clinical seizures in acquired epileptic aphasia (LKS) is 70-85%. In one third of patients, only a single episode of a seizure was recorded. The seizures typically appear between the ages of 4 and 10 and disappear before adulthood (around the age of 15).

Often, behavioral and neuropsychologic disturbances accompany the progression of LKS. Behavioral issues are seen in as many as 78% of all cases. Hyperactivity and a decreased attention span are observed in as many as 80% of patients as well as rage, aggression, and anxiety. These behavior patterns are considered secondary to the language impairment in LKS. Impaired short-term memory is a feature recorded in long-standing cases of acquired epileptic aphasia.

Cause

Most cases of LKS do not have a known cause.

Diagnosis

The syndrome can be difficult to diagnose and may be misdiagnosed as autism, pervasive developmental disorder, hearing impairment, learning disability, auditory/verbal processing disorder, attention deficit hyperactivity disorder, intellectual disability, childhood schizophrenia, or emotional/behavioral problems. An EEG (electroencephalogram) test is imperative to a diagnosis. Many cases of patients exhibiting LKS will show abnormal electrical brain activity in both the right and left hemispheres of the brain; this is exhibited frequently during sleep. Even though an abnormal EEG reading is common in LKS patients, a relationship has not been identified between EEG abnormalities and the presence and intensity of language problems. In many cases however, abnormalities in the EEG test has preceded language deterioration and improvement in the EEG tracing has preceded language improvement (this occurs in about half of all affected children). Many factors inhibit the reliability of the EEG data: neurologic deficits do not closely follow the maximal EEG changes in time.

The most effective way of confirming LKS is by obtaining overnight sleep EEGs, including EEGs in all stages of sleep. Many conditions like demyelination and brain tumors can be ruled out by using magnetic resonance imaging (MRI). In LKS, fluorodeoxyglucose (FDG) and positron emission tomography (PET) scanning can show decreased metabolism in one or both temporal lobes - hypermetabolism has been seen in patients with acquired epileptic aphasia.

Most cases of LKS do not have a known cause. Occasionally, the condition may be induced secondary to other diagnoses such as low-grade brain tumors, closed-head injury, neurocysticercosis, and demyelinating disease. Central Nervous System vasculitis may be associated with this condition as well.

Differential Diagnosis

The table below demonstrates the extensive and differential diagnosis of acquired epileptic aphasia along with Cognitive and Behavioral Regression:

Diagnosis	Deterioration	EEG Patterns
Autistic epileptiform regression	Expressive language, RL, S, verbal and nonverbal communication	Centrotemporal spikes
Autistic regression	Expressive language, RL, S, verbal and nonverbal communication	Normal
Acquired epileptic aphasia	RL, possibly behavioral	Left or right temporal or parietal spikes, possibly ESES
Acquired expressive epileptic aphasia	Expressive language, oromotor apraxia	Centrotemporal spikes
(ESES)	Expressive language, RL, possibly behavioral	ESES
Developmental dysphasia (developmental expressive language disease)	No; lack of expressive language acquisition	Temporal or parietal spikes
Disintegrative epileptiform disorder	Expressive language, RL, S, verbal and nonverbal communication, possibly behavioral	ESES
Stuttering	Expressive language, no verbal-auditory agnosia	Spike-and-wave discharges on the left temporocentral and frontal regions

Note: EEG = electroencephalographic; ESES = electrical status epilepticus of sleep; RL = receptive language; S = sociability

- Continuous spike and wave of slow-wave sleep (>85% of slow-wave sleep).

Treatment

Treatment for LKS usually consists of medications, such as anticonvulsants and corticosteroids (such as prednisone), and speech therapy, which should be started early. Some patients improve with the use of corticosteroids or adrenocorticotropin hormone (ACTH) which lead researches to believe that inflammation and vasospasm may play a role in some cases of acquired epileptic aphasia.

A controversial treatment option involves a surgical technique called multiple subpial transection in which multiple incisions are made through the cortex of the affected part of the brain beneath the pia mater, severing the axonal tracts in the subjacent white matter. The cortex is sliced in parallel lines to the midtemporal gyrus and perisylvian area to attenuate the spread of the epileptiform activity without causing cortical dysfunction. There is a study by Morrell *et al.* in which results were reported for 14 patients with acquired epileptic aphasia who underwent multiple subpial transections. Seven of the fourteen patients recovered age-appropriate speech and no longer required speech therapy. Another 4 of the 14 displayed improvement of speech and understanding instructions given verbally, but they still required speech therapy. Eleven patients had language dysfunction for two or more years. Another study by Sawhney *et al.* reported improvement in all three of their patients with acquired epileptic aphasia who underwent the same procedure.

Various hospitals contain programs designed to treat conditions such as LKS like the Children's Hospital Boston and its Augmentative Communication Program. It is known internationally for its work with children or adults who are non-speaking or severely impaired. Typically, a care team for children with LKS consists of a neurologist, a neuropsychologist, and a speech pathologist or audiologist. Some children with behavioral problems may also need to see a child psychologist and a psychopharmacologist. Speech therapy begins immediately at the time of diagnosis along with medical treatment that may include steroids and anti-epileptic or anti-convulsant medications.

Patient education has also proved to be helpful in treating LKS. Teaching them sign language is a helpful means of communication and if the child was able to read and write before the onset of LKS, that is extremely helpful too.

Prognosis

The prognosis for children with LKS varies. Some affected children may have a permanent severe language disorder, while others may regain much of their language abilities (although it may take months or years). In some cases, remission and relapse may occur. The prognosis is improved when the onset of the disorder is after age 6 and when speech therapy is started early. Seizures generally disappear by adulthood. Short-term remissions are not uncommon in LKS but they create difficulties in evaluating a patient's response to various therapeutic modalities.

The following table demonstrate the Long-Term Follow-up of Acquired Epileptic Aphasia across many different instrumental studies:.

Study	Number of Patients	Mean Follow-up, y	Number of Patients with Normal or Mild Language Problems
Soprano *et al.* (1994)	12	8	3
Mantovani and Landau (1980)	9	22	6
Paquier (1992)	6	8.1	3
Rossi (1999)	11	9.7	2
Robinson et all (2001)	18	5.6	3
Duran *et al.* (2009)	7	9.5	1
Total	63		18 (28.6%)

Lower rates of good outcomes have been reported, ranging between 14% to 50%. Duran *et al.* used 7 patients in his study (all males, aged 8–27 years of age) with LKS. On long-term followup, most of his patients did not demonstrate total epilepsy remission and language problems continued. Out of the seven patients, one reported a normal quality of life while the other six reported aphasia to be a substantial struggle. The Duran *et al.* study is one of few that features long-term follow up reports of LKS and utilizes EEG testing, MRIs, the Vineland Adaptive Behavior Scales, the Connor's Rating Scales-revised, and a Short-Form Health Survey to analyze its patients.

Globally, more than 200 cases of acquired epileptic aphasia have been described in the literature. Between 1957 and 1980, 81 cases of acquired epileptic aphasia were reported, with 100 cases generally being diagnosed every 10 years.

References

- Häggström, Mikael (2014). "Reference ranges for estradiol, progesterone, luteinizing hormone and follicle-stimulating hormone during the menstrual cycle". WikiJournal of Medicine. 1 (1). ISSN 2002-4436. doi:10.15347/wjm/2014.001
- Panayiotopoulos CP. The Epilepsies: Seizures, Syndromes and Management. Oxfordshire: Bladon Medical Publishing; 2005. ch. 6. ISBN 1-904218-34-2. PMID 20821848
- "Chapter 9 Benign childhood seizure susceptibility syndromes" (PDF). epilepsy society. Retrieved 26 April 2016
- Herzog AG (2008). "Catamenial epilepsy: Definition, prevalence, pathophysiology and treatment". Seizure. 17 (2): 151–9. PMID 18164632. doi:10.1016/j.seizure.2007.11.014
- Wirrell EC, Camfield PR, Gordon KE, Dooley JM, Camfield CS (1995). "Benign rolandic epilepsy: atypical features are very common". Journal of Child Neurology. 10 (6): 455–8. doi:10.1177/088307389501000606
- Røste LS, Taubøll E, Svalheim S, Gjerstad L (2008). "Does menopause affect the epilepsy?". Epilepsia. 17 (2): 172–5. PMID 18164217. doi:10.1016/j.seizure.2007.11.019
- Tütüncüoğlu S, Serdaroğlu G, Kadioğlu B (October 2002). "Landau-Kleffner syndrome beginning with stuttering: case report". Journal of Child Neurology. 17 (10): 785–8. PMID 12546439. doi:10.1177/08830738020170101808
- Temkin, Owsei (March 1, 1994) [First published 1945, Revised 1971]. The Falling Sickness (2nd Revised ed.). Baltimore: Johns Hopkins University Press. ISBN 978-0-8018-4849-0
- Caraballo R, Cersosimo R, Fejerman N (June 2007). "Panayiotopoulos syndrome: a prospective study of 192 patients". Epilepsia. 48 (6): 1054–61. PMID 17442007. doi:10.1111/j.1528-1167.2007.01085.x

4

Epileptic Seizure: An Integrated Study

Epileptic seizures occur when the neuronal activity of the brain increases to an abnormal level, causing momentary loss of consciousness and uncontrollable jerking and muscle spasms. Epilepsy causes a paroxysmal depolarizing shift, with brain neurons firing in an uncoordinated manner. The aspects elucidated in this chapter are of vital importance, and provide a better understanding of epilepsy.

Epileptic Seizure

An epileptic seizure, also known as an epileptic fit, seizure or fit, is a brief episode of signs or symptoms due to abnormal excessive or synchronous neuronal activity in the brain. The outward effect can vary from uncontrolled jerking movement (tonic-clonic seizure) to as subtle as a momentary loss of awareness (absence seizure). Diseases of the brain characterized by an enduring predisposition to generate epileptic seizures are collectively called epilepsy.

Seizures can also occur in people who do not have epilepsy for various reasons including brain trauma, drug use, elevated body temperature, low blood sugar and low levels of oxygen. Additionally, there are a number of conditions that look like epileptic seizures but are not.

A first seizure generally does not require long term treatment with anti-seizure medications unless there is a specific problem on either electroencephalogram or brain imaging.

5–10% of people who live to 80 years old have at least one epileptic seizure and the chance of experiencing a second seizure is between 40% and 50%. About 50% of patients with an unprovoked apparent "first seizure" have had other minor seizures, so their diagnosis is epilepsy. Epilepsy affects about 1% of the population currently and affected about 4% of the population at some point in time. Most of those affected—nearly 80%—live in developing countries.

Signs and Symptoms

The signs and symptoms of seizures vary depending on the type. The most common type of seizure is convulsive (60%). Two-thirds of these begin as focal seizures and become generalized while one third begin as generalized seizures. The remaining 40% of seizures are non-convulsive, an example of which is absence seizure.

Focal Seizures

Focal seizures are often preceded by certain experiences, known as an aura. These may include: sensory, visual, psychic, autonomic, olfactory or motor phenomena.

In a complex partial seizure a person may appear confused or dazed and can not respond to questions or direction. Focal seizure may become generalized.

Jerking activity may start in a specific muscle group and spread to surrounding muscle groups—known as a *Jacksonian march*. Unusual activities that are not consciously created may occur. These are known as automatisms and include simple activities like smacking of the lips or more complex activities such as attempts to pick something up.

Generalized Seizures

There are six main types of generalized seizures: tonic-clonic, tonic, clonic, myoclonic, absence, and atonic seizures. They all involve a loss of consciousness and typically happen without warning.

- Tonic-clonic seizures present with a contraction of the limbs followed by their extension, along with arching of the back for 10–30 seconds. A cry may be heard due to contraction of the chest muscles. The limbs then begin to shake in unison. After the shaking has stopped it may take 10–30 minutes for the person to return to normal.
- Tonic seizures produce constant contractions of the muscles. The person may turn blue if breathing is impaired.
- Clonic seizures involve shaking of the limbs in unison.
- Myoclonic seizures involve spasms of muscles in either a few areas or generalized through the body.
- Absence seizures can be subtle, with only a slight turn of the head or eye blinking. The person often does not fall over and may return to normal right after the seizure ends, though there may also be a period of post-ictal disorientation.
- Atonic seizures involve the loss of muscle activity for greater than one second. This typically occurs bilaterally (on both sides of the body).

Duration

A seizure can last from a few seconds to more than five minutes, at which point it is known as status epilepticus. Most tonic-clonic seizures last less than two or three minutes. Absence seizures are usually around 10 seconds in duration.

Postictal

After the active portion of a seizure, there is typically a period of confusion called the *postictal period* before a normal level of consciousness returns. This usually lasts 3 to 15 minutes but may last for hours. Other common symptoms include: feeling tired, headache, difficulty speaking, and abnormal behavior. Psychosis after a seizure is relatively common, occurring in between 6 and 10% of people. Often people do not remember what occurred during this time.

Causes

Seizures have a number of causes. Of those with seizure about 25% have epilepsy. A number of conditions are associated with seizures but are not epilepsy including: most febrile seizures and those that occur around an acute infection, stroke, or toxicity. These seizures are known as “acute symptomatic” or “provoked” seizures and are part of the seizure-related disorders. In many the cause is unknown.

Different causes of seizures are common in certain age groups.

- During the neonatal period and early infancy the most common causes include hypoxic ischemic encephalopathy, central nervous system (CNS) infections, trauma, congenital CNS abnormalities, and metabolic disorders.
- The most frequent cause of seizures in children is febrile seizures, which happen in 2–5% of children between the ages of six months and five years.
- During childhood, well-defined epilepsy syndromes are generally seen.
- In adolescence and young adulthood, non-compliance with the medication regimen and sleep deprivation are potential triggers.
- Pregnancy and labor and childbirth, and the post-partum, or post-natal period (after birth) can be at-risk times, especially if there are certain complications like pre-eclampsia.
- During adulthood, the likely causes are alcohol related, strokes, trauma, CNS infections, and brain tumors.
- In older adults, cerebrovascular disease is a very common cause. Other causes are CNS tumors, head trauma, and other degenerative diseases that are common in the older age group, such as dementia.

Metabolic

Dehydration can trigger epileptic seizures if it is severe enough. A number of disorders including: low blood sugar, low blood sodium, hyperosmolar nonketotic hyperglycemia, high blood sodium, low blood calcium and high blood urea levels may cause seizures. As may hepatic encephalopathy and the genetic disorder porphyria.

Mass Lesions

- cavernoma or cavernous malformation is a treatable medical condition that can cause seizures, headaches, and brain hemorrhages.
- arteriovenous malformation (AVM) is a treatable medical condition that can cause seizures, headaches, and brain hemorrhages.
- space-occupying lesions in the brain (abscesses, tumours). In people with brain tumours, the frequency of epilepsy depends on the location of the tumor in the cortical region.

Medications

Both medication and drug overdoses can result in seizures, as may certain medication and drug withdrawal. Common drugs involved include: antidepressants, antipsychotics, cocaine, insulin, and the local anaesthetic lidocaine. Difficulties with withdrawal seizures commonly occurs after prolonged alcohol or sedative use, a condition known as delerium tremens.

Infections

- Infection with the pork tapeworm, which can cause neurocysticercosis, is the cause of up to half of epilepsy cases in areas of the world where the parasite is common
- parasitic infections such as cerebral malaria
- infection, such as encephalitis or meningitis

Other

Seizures may occur as a result of high blood pressure, known as hypertensive encephalopathy, or in pregnancy as eclampsia when accompanied by either seizures or a decreased level of consciousness. Very high body temperatures may also be a cause. Typically this requires a temperature greater than 42 °C (107.6 °F).

- Head injury may cause non-epileptic post-traumatic seizures or post-traumatic epilepsy
- About 3.5 to 5.5% of people with celiac disease also have seizures
- Seizures in a person with a shunt may indicate failure
- Hemorrhagic stroke can occasionally present with seizures, embolic strokes generally do not (though epilepsy is a common later complication); cerebral venous sinus thrombosis, a rare type of stroke, is more likely to be accompanied by seizures than other types of stroke
- multiple sclerosis may cause seizures

Electroconvulsive therapy (ECT) deliberately sets out to induce a seizure for the treatment of major depression.

Mechanism

Normally brain electrical activity is non synchronous. In epileptic seizures, due to problems within the brain, a group of neurons begin firing in an abnormal, excessive, and synchronized manner. This results in a wave of depolarization known as a paroxysmal depolarizing shift.

Normally after an excitatory neuron fires it becomes more resistant to firing for a period of time. This is due in part from the effect of inhibitory neurons, electrical changes within the excitatory neuron, and the negative effects of adenosine. In epilepsy the resistance of excitatory neurons to fire during this period is decreased. This may occur due to changes in ion channels or inhibitory neurons not functioning properly. This then results in a specific area from which seizures may develop, known as a "seizure focus". Following an injury to the brain, another mechanism of epilepsy may be the up regulation of excitatory circuits or down regulation of inhibitory circuits. These secondary epilepsies occur through processes known as epileptogenesis. Failure of the blood–brain barrier may also be a causal mechanism.

Focal seizures begin in one hemisphere of the brain while generalized seizures begin in both hemispheres. Some types of seizures may change brain structure, while others appear to have little effect. Gliosis, neuronal loss, and atrophy of specific areas of the brain are linked to epilepsy but it is unclear if epilepsy causes these changes or if these changes result in epilepsy.

Seizure activity may be propagated through the brain's endogenous electrical fields.

Diagnosis

It is important to distinguish primary seizures from secondary causes. Depending on the presumed cause blood tests and/or lumbar puncture may be useful. Hypoglycemia may cause seizures and should be ruled out. An electroencephalogram and brain imaging with CT scan or MRI scan is recommended in the work-up of seizures not associated with a fever.

Classification

Seizure types are organized by whether the source of the seizure is localized (focal seizures) or distributed (generalized seizures) within the brain. Generalized seizures are divided according to the effect on the body and include tonic-clonic (grand mal), absence (petit mal), myoclonic, clonic, tonic, and atonic seizures. Some seizures such as epileptic spasms are of an unknown type.

Focal seizures (previously called *partial seizures*) are divided into simple partial or complex partial seizure. Current practice no longer recommends this, and instead prefers to describe what occurs during a seizure.

Physical Examination

Most people are in a postictal state (drowsy or confused) following a seizure. They may show signs of other injuries. A bite mark on the side of the tongue helps confirm a seizure when present, but only a third of people who have had a seizure have such a bite.

Tests

An electroencephalography is only recommended in those who likely had an epileptic seizure and may help determine the type of seizure or syndrome present. In children it is typically only needed after a second seizure. It cannot be used to rule out the diagnosis and may be falsely positive in those without the disease. In certain situations it may be useful to prefer the EEG while sleeping or sleep deprived.

Diagnostic imaging by CT scan and MRI is recommended after a first non-febrile seizure to detect structural problems inside the brain. MRI is generally a better imaging test except when intracranial bleeding is suspected. Imaging may be done at a later point in time in those who return to their normal selves while in the emergency room. If a person has a previous diagnosis of epilepsy with previous imaging repeat imaging is not usually needed with subsequent seizures.

In adults, testing electrolytes, blood glucose and calcium levels is important to rule these out as causes, as is an electrocardiogram. A lumbar puncture may be useful to diagnose a central nervous system infection but is not routinely needed. Routine antiseizure medical levels in the blood are not required in adults or children. In children additional tests may be required.

A high blood prolactin level within the first 20 minutes following a seizure may be useful to confirm an epileptic seizure as opposed to psychogenic non-epileptic seizure. Serum prolactin level is less useful for detecting partial seizures. If it is normal an epileptic seizure is still possible and a serum prolactin does not separate epileptic seizures from syncope. It is not recommended as a routine part of diagnosis epilepsy.

Differential Diagnosis

Differentiating an epileptic seizure from other conditions such as syncope can be difficult. Other possible conditions that can mimic a seizure include: decerebrate posturing, psychogenic seizures, tetanus, dystonia, migraine headaches, and strychnine poisoning. In addition, 5% of people with a positive tilt table test may have seizure-like activity that seems to be due to cerebral hypoxia. Convulsions may occur due to psychological reasons and this is known as a psychogenic non-epileptic seizure. Non-epileptic seizures may also occur due to a number of other reasons.

Prevention

A number of measures have been attempted to prevent seizures in those at risk. Following traumatic brain injury anticonvulsants decrease the risk of early seizures but not late seizures.

In those with a history of febrile seizures, medications (both antipyretics and anticonvulsants) have not been found effective for prevention. Some, in fact, may cause harm.

There is no clear evidence that antiepileptic drugs are effective or not effective at preventing seizures following a craniotomy, following subdural hematoma, after a stroke, or after subarachnoid haemorrhage, for both people who have had a previous seizure, and those who have not.

Management

Potentially sharp or dangerous objects should be moved from the area around a person experiencing a seizure, so that the individual is not hurt. After the seizure if the person is not fully conscious and alert, they should be placed in the recovery position. A seizure longer than five minutes is a medical emergency known as status epilepticus. Contrary to a common misconception, bystanders should not attempt to force objects into the mouth of the person suffering a seizure, as doing so may cause injury to the teeth and gums.

Medication

The first line treatment of choice for someone who is actively seizing is a benzodiazepine, most guidelines recommend lorazepam. This may be repeated if there is no effect after 10 minutes. If there is no effect after two doses, barbiturates or propofol may be used. Benzodiazepines given by a non-intravenous route appear to be better than those given by intravenous as the intravenous takes time to start.

Ongoing anti-epileptic medications are not typically recommended after a first seizure except in those with structural lesions in the brain. They are generally recommended after a second one has occurred. Approximately 70% of people can obtain full control with continuous use of medication. Typically one type of anticonvulsant is preferred. Following a first seizure, while immediate treatment with an anti-seizure drug lowers the probability of seizure recurrence up to five years it does not change the risk of death and there are potential side effects.

In seizures related to toxins, up to two doses of benzodiazepines should be used. If this is not effective pyridoxine is recommended. Phenytoin should generally not be used.

There is a lack of evidence for preventative anti epileptic medications in the management of seizures, primary or secondary to intracranial venous thrombosis.

Other

Helmets may be used to provide protection to the head during a seizure. Some claim that seizure response dogs, a form of service dog, can predict seizures. Evidence for this, however, is poor. At present there is not enough evidence to support the use of cannabis for the management of seizures, although this is an ongoing area of research. There is tentative evidence that a ketogenic diet may help in those who have epilepsy and is reasonable in those who do not improve following typical treatments.

Prognosis

Following a first seizure, the risk of more seizures in the next two years is 40%–50%. The greatest predictors of more seizures are problems either on the electroencephalogram or on imaging of the brain. In adults, after 6 months of being seizure-free after a first seizure, the risk of a subsequent seizure in the next year is less than 20% regardless of treatment. Up to 7% of seizures that present to the emergency department (ER) are in status epilepticus. In those with a status epilepticus, mortality is between 10% and 40%. Those who have a seizure that is provoked (occurring close in time to an acute brain event or toxic exposure) have a low risk of re-occurrence, but have a higher risk of death compared to those with epilepsy.

Epidemiology

5–10% of people who live to 80 years old have at least one epileptic seizure and the chance of experiencing a second seizure is between 40% and 50%. About 0.7% in the general population of the United States go to an emergency department after a seizure in a given year, 7% of them with status epilepticus. Known epilepsy though is an uncommon cause of seizures in the emergency department, accounting for a minority of seizure-related visits. About 50% of patients with an unprovoked apparent "first seizure" have had other minor seizures, so their diagnosis is epilepsy.

History

The word epilepsy derives from the Greek word for "attack." Seizures were long viewed as an otherworldly condition and this view was seen by Hippocrates (400 BC) as treating it as a *sacred disease* which he wrote about and concluded that it had natural causes just as other diseases did.In the mid 1800s the first anti seizure medication, bromide, was introduced.

Following standardization proposals devised by Henri Gastaut and published in 1970, terms such as "petit mal", "grand mal", "Jacksonian", "psychomotor", and "temporal-lobe seizure" have fallen into disuse.

Society and Culture

Economics

Seizures result in direct economic costs of about one billion dollars in the United States. Epilepsy results in economic costs in Europe of around 15.5 billion Euros in 2004. In India, epilepsy is estimated to result in costs of 1.7 billion USD or 0.5% of the GDP. They make up about 1% of emergency department visits (2% for emergency departments for children) in the United States.

Driving

Many areas of the world require a minimum of six months from the last seizure before people can drive a vehicle.

Seizure Types

Seizure types most commonly follow the classification proposed by the International League Against Epilepsy (ILAE) in 1981. Distinguishing between seizure types is important since different types of seizure may have different causes, outcomes and treatments.

International Classification of Seizure Types (1981)

This classification is based on observation (clinical and EEG) rather than the underlying pathophysiology or anatomy.

I. Focal seizures (Older term: partial seizures)

A. Simple partial seizures – consciousness is not impaired

1. With motor signs
2. With sensory symptoms
3. With autonomic symptoms or signs
4. With psychic symptoms

B. Complex partial seizures – consciousness is impaired (Older terms: temporal lobe or psychomotor seizures)

1. Simple partial onset, followed by impairment of consciousness
2. With impairment of consciousness at onset

C. Partial seizures evolving to secondarily generalized seizures

1. Simple partial seizures evolving to generalized seizures

2. Complex partial seizures evolving to generalized seizures

3. Simple partial seizures evolving to complex partial seizures evolving to generalized seizures

II. Generalized seizures

A. Absence seizures (Older term: petit mal)

1. Typical absence seizures

2. Atypical absence seizures

B. Myoclonic seizures

C. Clonic seizures

D. Tonic seizures,

E. Tonic–clonic seizures (Older term: grand mal)

F. Atonic seizures

III. Unclassified epileptic seizures

In terms of their origin within the brain, seizures may be described as either *partial* (focal) or *generalized*. Partial seizures only involve a localized part of the brain, whereas generalized seizures involve the whole of both hemispheres. The term 'secondary generalisation' may be used to describe a partial seizure that later spreads to the whole of the cortex and becomes generalized.

Whilst most seizures can be neatly split into partial and generalized, there exists some that don't fit. For example: the seizure may be generalized only within one hemisphere. Alternatively there may be many focal points (*multifocal seizures*) that are distributed in a symmetrical or asymmetrical pattern.

Partial Seizures

Partial seizures may be further subdivided into both *simple* and *complex* seizures. This refers to the effect of such a seizure on consciousness; simple seizures cause no interruption to consciousness (although they may cause sensory distortions or other sensations), whereas complex seizures interrupt consciousness to varying degrees. This does not necessarily mean that the person experiencing this sort of seizure will fall unconscious (like fainting). For example, a complex partial seizure may involve the unconscious repetition of simple actions, gestures or verbal utterances, or simply a blank stare and apparent unawareness of the occurrence of the seizure, followed by no memory of the seizure. Other patients may report a feeling of tunnel vision or dissociation, which represents a diminishment of awareness without full loss of consciousness. Still other patients can perform complicated actions, such as travel or shopping, while in the midst of a complex partial seizure.

The effects of partial seizures can be quite dependent on the area of the brain in which they are active. For example, a partial seizure in areas involved in perception may cause a particular sensory experience (for example, the perception of a scent, music or flashes of light) whereas, when centred in the motor cortex, a partial seizure might cause movement in particular groups of muscles. This type of seizure may also produce particular thoughts or internal visual images or even experiences which may be distinct but not easily described. Seizures centered on the temporal lobes may produce brief mystical or ecstatic experiences in some people; these are known as ecstatic seizures. They may result in a misdiagnosis of psychosis or schizophrenia, if other symptoms of seizure are disregarded and other tests are not performed. Unfortunately for those with epilepsy, anti-psychotic medications prescribed without anticonvulsants in this case can actually lower the seizure threshold further and worsen the symptoms.

When the effects of a partial seizure appear as a 'warning sign' before a larger seizure, they are known as an aura: it is frequently the case that a partial seizure will spread to other parts of the brain and eventually become generalized, resulting in a tonic-clonic convulsion. The subjective experience of an aura, like other partial seizures, will tend to reflect the function of the affected part of the brain.

Generalized Seizures

Primarily generalized seizures can be sub-classified into a number of categories, depending on their behavioural effects:

- *Absence seizures* involve an interruption to consciousness where the person experiencing the seizure seems to become vacant and unresponsive for a short period of time (usually up to 30 seconds). Slight muscle twitching may occur.
- *Myoclonic seizures* involve an extremely brief (< 0.1 second) muscle contraction and can result in jerky movements of muscles or muscle groups.
- *Clonic seizures* are myoclonus that are regularly repeating at a rate typically of 2-3 per second. In some cases, the length varies.
- *Tonic–clonic seizures* involve an initial contraction of the muscles (*tonic phase*) which may involve tongue biting, urinary incontinence and the absence of breathing. This is followed by rhythmic muscle contractions (*clonic phase*). This type of seizure is usually what is referred to when the term 'epileptic fit' is used colloquially.

- *Atonic seizures* involve the loss of muscle tone, causing the person to fall to the ground. These are sometimes called 'drop attacks' but should be distinguished from similar looking attacks that may occur in cataplexy.

Continuous Seizures

Status epilepticus refers to continuous seizure activity with no recovery between successive seizures. A tonic-clonic seizure lasting longer than 5 minutes (or two minutes longer than a given person's usual seizures) is considered a medical emergency. Benzodiazepines are most commonly used to relieve the seizure activity.

Epilepsia partialis continua is a rare type of focal motor seizure (hands and face) which recurs every few seconds or minutes for extended periods (days or years). It is usually due to strokes in adults and focal cortical inflammatory processes in children (Rasmussen's encephalitis), possibly caused by chronic viral infections or autoimmune processes.

Future Classifications

In 1997, the ILAE began work on revising the classification of seizures, epilepsies and epileptic syndromes. This revision remains in gestation and has not superseded the 1981 classification.

Proposed changes to terminology include:

- Replace *partial* with the older term *focal* to describe seizures that originate in one part of the brain (though not necessarily a small or well defined area). The word partial was regarded as ambiguous.
- Drop the terms *simple partial* and *complex partial* - grouping based on the effect to consciousness is no longer regarded as useful.
- Replace *cryptogenic* with *probably symptomatic.*

The hierarchy presented has the structure:

Self limiting seizure types

Generalized seizures

- Tonic-clonic seizures
- Clonic seizures
- Typical absence seizures
- Atypical absence seizures
- Myoclonic absence seizures
- Tonic seizures
- Spasms
- Myoclonic seizures
- Massive bilateral myoclonus
- Eyelid myoclonia
- Myoclonic atonic seizures
- Negative myoclonus
- Atonic seizures
- Reflex seizures in generalized epilepsy syndromes
- Seizures of the posterior neocortex
- Neocortical temporal lobe seizures

Focal seizures

- Focal sensory seizures
- Focal motor seizures
- Gelastic seizures
- Hemiclonic seizures
- Secondarily generalized seizures
- Reflex seizures in focal epilepsy syndromes

Continuous seizure types

Generalized status epilepticus

- Generalized tonic-clonic status epilepticus
- Clonic status epilepticus
- Absence status epilepticus
- Tonic status epilepticus
- Myoclonic status epilepticus

Focal status epilepticus

- Epilepsia partialis continua of Kojevnikov
- Aura continua
- Limbic status epilepticus
- Hemiconvulsive status with hemiparesis

Earlier Classifications

The 1981 classification revised the 1970 ILAE system devised by Henri Gastaut. A significant difference was the distinction between simple and complex partial seizures. In the 1970 classification, the distinction was whether the symptoms involved elementary sensory or motor functions (simple) or whether "higher functions" were involved (complex). This was changed to consider whether consciousness was fully retained or not. As a result, studies that group patients according to these classifications are not directly comparable from one generation to another. The 1970 classification was important for standardising the modern terms for many seizure types. Prior to this, terms such as *petit mal*, *grand mal*, *Jacksonian*, *psychomotor* and *temporal-lobe* seizures were used.

The earliest classification of seizures can be attributed to Babylonian scholars who inscribed their medical knowledge into stone tablets known as the *Sakikku* (meaning *All Diseases*). This dates from the reign of the Babylonian king Adad-apla-iddina of the Second Dynasty of Isin - estimated to be between 1067 and 1046 BC. Many types of seizures are described, each attributed to a certain demon or departed spirit and given a prognosis.

Focal Seizure

Focal seizures (also called partial seizures and localized seizures) are seizures which affect initially only one hemisphere of the brain. The brain is divided into two hemispheres, each consisting of four lobes – the frontal, temporal, parietal and occipital lobes. In partial seizures the seizure is generated in and affects just one part of the brain – the whole hemisphere or part of a lobe. Symptoms will vary according to where the seizure occurs. In the frontal lobe symptoms may include a wave-like sensation in the head; in the temporal lobe, a feeling of déjà vu; in the parietal lobe, a numbness or tingling; and in the occipital lobe, visual disturbance or hallucination.

Focal seizures are split into two main categories; simple focal seizures and complex focal seizures.

In simple focal seizures a small part of one of the lobes may be affected and the person remains conscious. This will often be a precursor to a larger seizure such as a complex partial seizure. When this is the case, the simple partial seizure is usually called an aura.

A complex focal seizure affects a larger part of the hemisphere than a simple partial seizure and the person may lose consciousness.

If a focal seizure spreads from one hemisphere to the other side of the brain, this will give rise to a secondarily generalised seizure. The person will become unconscious and may well have a tonic clonic seizure. When people have multiple focal seizures they generally have a condition known as temporal lobe epilepsy.

Simple Focal Seizure

Simple focal seizures are seizures which affect only a small region of the brain, often the temporal lobes or hippocampi. People who have simple partial seizures retain consciousness. Simple partial seizures often precede larger seizures, where the abnormal electrical activity spreads to a larger area of (or all of) the brain, usually resulting in a complex partial seizure or a tonic-clonic seizure. In this case they are often known as an aura.

Presentation

Simple partial seizures are a very subjective experience, and the symptoms of a simple partial seizure vary greatly between people. This is due to the varying locations of the brain the seizures originate in e.g.: Rolandic. A simple partial seizure may go unnoticed by others or shrugged off by the sufferer as merely a "funny turn." Simple partial seizures usually start suddenly and are very brief, typically lasting 60 to 120 seconds.

While awake some common symptoms of simple partial seizures are:

- preserved consciousness
- sudden and inexplicable feelings of fear, anger, sadness, happiness or nausea
- sensations of falling or movement
- experiencing of unusual feelings or sensations

- altered sense of hearing, smelling, tasting, seeing, and tactile perception (sensory illusions or hallucinations), or feeling as though the environment is not real (derealization) or dissociation from the environment or self (depersonalization)
- a sense of spatial distortion—things close by may appear to be at a distance
- déjà vu (familiarity) or jamais vu (unfamiliarity)
- laboured speech or inability to speak at all
- usually the event is remembered in detail

When the seizure occurs during sleep, the person will often become semi-conscious and act out a dream they were having while engaging with the real environment as normal. Objects and people usually appear normal or only slightly distorted to them, and will be able to communicate with them on an otherwise normal level. However, since the person is still acting in the dream-like state from which they woke, they will assimilate any hallucinations or delusions into their communication, often speaking to a hallucinatory person or speaking of events or thoughts normally pertaining to the dream they were having or other hallucination.

While asleep symptoms include:

- onset usually in REM sleep
- dream like state
- appearance of full consciousness
- hallucinations or delusions
- behavior or visions typical in dreams
- ability to engage with the environment and other people as in full consciousness, though often behaving abnormally, erratically, or failing to be coherent
- complete amnesia or assimilating the memory as though it was a normal dream on regaining full consciousness

Although hallucinations may occur during simple partial seizures they are differentiated from psychotic symptoms by the fact that the person is usually aware that the hallucinations are not real.

Jacksonian March

Jacksonian march or Jacksonian seizure is a phenomenon where a simple partial seizure spreads from the distal part of the limb toward the ipsilateral face (on same side of body). They involve a progression of the location of the seizure in the brain, which leads to a “march” of the motor presentation of symptoms.

Jacksonian seizures are initiated with abnormal electrical activity within the primary motor cortex. They are unique in that they travel through the primary motor cortex in succession, affecting the corresponding muscles, often beginning with the fingers. This is felt as a tingling sensation, or a feeling of waves through the fingers when touched together. It then affects the hand and moves on to more proximal areas on the same side of body. Symptoms often associated with a Jacksonian seizure are sudden head and eye movements, tingling, numbness, smacking of the lips, and sudden muscle contractions. Most of the time any one of these actions can be seen as normal movements, without being associated with the seizure occurring. They occur at no particular moment and last only briefly. They may result in secondary generalized seizure involving both hemispheres. They can also start at the feet, manifesting as tingling or pins and needles, and there are painful cramps in the foot muscles, due to the signals from the brain. Because it is a partial seizure, the postictal state is of normal consciousness.

Eponym

These seizures are named after their discoverer, John Hughlings Jackson, an English neurologist, whose studies led to the discovery of the seizures' initiation point (in the primary motor cortex) in 1863.

Complex Focal Seizure

A complex focal seizure is an epileptic seizure that is associated with unilateral cerebral hemisphere involvement and causes impairment of awareness or responsiveness, i.e. alteration of consciousness.

Presentation

Complex focal seizures are often preceded by a seizure aura. The seizure aura is a simple partial seizure. The aura may manifest itself as a feeling of déjà vu, jamais vu, fear, euphoria or depersonalization. The seizure aura might also occur as a visual disturbance, such as tunnel vision or a change in the perceived size of objects. Once consciousness is impaired, the person may display automatisms such as lip smacking, chewing or swallowing. There may also be loss of memory (amnesia) surrounding the seizural event. The person may still be able to perform routine tasks such as walking, although such movements are not purposeful or planned. Witnesses may not recognize that anything is wrong.

Complex partial seizures might arise from any lobe of the brain. Complex partial seizures most commonly arise from the mesial temporal lobe, particularly the amygdala, hippocampus, and neocortical regions. A common associated brain abnormality is mesial temporal sclerosis. Mesial temporal sclerosis is a specific pattern of hippocampal neuronal loss accompanied by hippocampal gliosis and atrophy. Complex partial seizures occur when excessive and synchronous electrical brain activity causes impaired awareness and responsiveness. The abnormal electrical activity might spread to the rest of the brain and cause a secondary generalized tonic–clonic seizure.

Absence Seizure

Absence seizures are one of several kinds of seizures. These seizures are sometimes referred to as petit mal seizures (from the French for "little illness", a term dating from the late 18th century). Absence seizures are characterized by a brief loss and return of consciousness, generally not followed by a period of lethargy (without a notable post-ictal state).

Signs and Symptoms

The clinical manifestations of absence seizures vary significantly among patients. Impairment of consciousness is the essential symptom, and may be the only clinical symptom, but this can be combined with other manifestations. The hallmark of the absence seizures is abrupt and sudden-onset impairment of consciousness, interruption of ongoing activities, a blank stare, possibly a brief upward rotation of the eyes. If the patient is speaking, speech is slowed or interrupted; if walking, they stand transfixed; if eating, the food will stop on its way to the mouth. Usually, the patient will be unresponsive when addressed. In some cases, attacks are aborted when the patient is called. The attack lasts from a few seconds to half a minute, and evaporates as rapidly as it commenced. Absence seizures generally are not followed by a period of disorientation or lethargy (post-ictal state), in contrast to the majority of seizure disorders.

1. Absence with impairment of consciousness only as per the above description.
2. Absence with mild clonic components. Here the onset of the attack is indistinguishable from the above, but clonic components may occur in the eyelids, at the corner of the mouth, or in other muscle groups which may vary in severity from almost imperceptible movements to generalised myoclonic jerks. Objects held in the hand may be dropped.
3. Absence with atonic components. Here there may be a diminution in tone of muscles subserving posture as well as in the limbs leading to dropping of the head, occasionally slumping of the trunk, dropping of the arms, and relaxation of the grip. Rarely tone is sufficiently diminished to cause this person to fall.
4. Absence with tonic components. Here during the attack tonic muscular contraction may occur, leading to increase in muscle tone which may affect the extensor muscles or the flexor muscles symmetrically or asymmetrically. If the patient is standing, the head may be drawn backward and the trunk may arch. This may lead to retropulsion, which may cause eyelids to twitch rapidly, eyes may jerk upwards or the patients head may rock back and forth slowly, as if nodding. The head may tonically draw to one or another side.

5. Absence with automatisms. Purposeful or quasipurposeful movements occurring in the absence of awareness during an absence attack are frequent and may range from lip licking and swallowing to clothes fumbling or aimless walking. If spoken to, the patient may grunt, and when touched or tickled may rub the site. Automatisms are quite elaborate and may consist of combinations of the above described movements or may be so simple as to be missed by casual observation.
6. Absence with autonomic components. These may be pallor, and less frequently flushing, sweating, dilatation of pupils and incontinence of urine.

Mixed forms of absence frequently occur. These seizures can happen a few times a day or in some cases hundreds of times a day, to the point that the person cannot concentrate in school or in other situations requiring sustained, concentrated attention.

Risk Factors

Typical absences are easily induced by hyperventilation in more than 90% of people with typical absences. This is a reliable test for the diagnosis of absence seizures: a patient suspected of typical absences should be asked to overbreathe for 3 minutes, counting their breaths. Intermittent photic stimulation may precipitate or facilitate absence seizures; eyelid myoclonia is a common clinical feature.

A specific mechanism difference exists in absence seizures in that T-type Ca++ channels are believed to be involved. Ethosuximide is specific for these channels and thus it is not effective for treating other types of seizure. Valproate and gabapentin (among others) have multiple mechanisms of action including blockade of T-type Ca++ channels and are useful in treating multiple seizure types. Gabapentin can aggravate absence seizures.

Diagnosis

The primary diagnostic test for absence seizures is EEG. However, brain scans such as by an MRI can help rule out other diseases, such as a stroke or a brain tumor.

During electroencephalography, hyperventilation can be used to provoke these seizures. Ambulatory EEG monitoring over 24 hours can quantify the number of seizures per day and their most likely times of occurrence.

Absence seizures are brief (usually less than 20 seconds) generalized epileptic seizures of sudden onset and termination. When someone experiences an absence seizure they are often unaware of their episode. Those most susceptible to this are children, and the first episode usually occurs between 4–12 years old. It is very rare that someone older will experience their first absence seizure. Episodes of absence seizures can often be mistaken for inattentiveness when misdiagnosed, and can occur 50-100 times a day. They can be so difficult to detect that some people may go months or years before being given a proper diagnosis. There are no known before or after effects of absence seizures.

Absence seizures have two essential components:

- Clinical - the impairment of consciousness (absence)
- Electroencephalography - an (EEG) shows generalized spike-and-slow wave discharges

Absence seizures are broadly divided into typical and atypical types:

- Typical absence seizures usually occur in the context of idiopathic generalised epilepsies and an EEG shows fast >2.5 Hz generalised spike-wave discharges. The prefix "typical" is to differentiate them from atypical absences rather than to characterise them as "classical" or characteristic of any particular syndrome.
- Atypical absence seizures:
    - Occur only in the context of mainly severe symptomatic or cryptogenic epilepsies of children with learning difficulties who also suffer from frequent seizures of other types, such as atonic, tonic and myoclonic.
    - Onset and termination is not so abrupt and changes in tone are more pronounced.
    - Ictal - EEG is of slow (less than 2.5 Hz) spike and slow wave. The discharge is heterogeneous, often asymmetrical and may include irregular spike and slow wave complexes, fast and other paroxysmal activity. Background interictal EEG is usually abnormal.

Syndromes

These syndromes are childhood absence epilepsy, epilepsy with myoclonic absences, juvenile absence epilepsy and juvenile myoclonic epilepsy. Other proposed syndromes are Jeavons syndrome (eyelid myoclonia with absences), and genetic generalised epilepsy with phantom absences.

These types of seizures are also known to occur to patients suffering with porphyria and can be triggered by stress or other porphyrin-inducing factors.

Treatment

Treatment of patients with absence seizures only is mainly with valproic acid or ethosuximide, which are of equal efficacy controlling absences in around 75% of patients. Lamotrigine monotherapy is less effective, with nearly half of the patients becoming seizure free. This view has been recently confirmed by Glauser et al. (2010), who studied the effects of ethosuximide, valproic acid, and lamotrigine in children with newly diagnosed childhood absence epilepsy. Drug dosages were incrementally increased until the child was free of seizures, the maximal allowable dose was reached, or a criterion indicating treatment failure was met. The primary outcome was freedom from treatment failure after 16 weeks of therapy; the secondary outcome was attentional dysfunction. After 16 weeks of therapy, the freedom-from-failure rates for ethosuximide and valproic acid were similar and were higher than the rate for lamotrigine. There were no significant differences between the three drugs with regard to discontinuation because of adverse events. Attentional dysfunction was more common with valproic acid than with ethosuximide. If monotherapy fails or unacceptable adverse reactions appear, replacement of one by another of the three antiepileptic drugs is the alternative. Adding small doses of lamotrigine to sodium valproate may be the best combination in resistant cases.

While ethosuximide is effective in treating only absence seizures, valproic acid is effective in treating multiple seizure types including tonic-clonic seizure and partial seizure, as such it may be a better choice if a patient is exhibiting multiple types of seizures. Similarly, lamotrigine treats multiple seizure types including partial seizures and generalized seizures, therefore it is also an option for patients with multiple seizure types. Clonazepam (Klonopin, Rivotril) is effective in the short term but is not generally recommended for treatment of absence seizure because of the rapid development of tolerance and high frequency of side effects.

Contraindicated Drugs

Carbamazepine, vigabatrin, and tiagabine are contraindicated in the treatment of absence seizures, irrespective of cause and severity. This is based on clinical and experimental evidence. In particular, the GABA agonists vigabatrin and tiagabine are used to induce, not to treat, absence seizures and absence status epilepticus. Similarly, oxcarbazepine, phenytoin, phenobarbital, gabapentin, and pregabalin should not be used in the treatment of absence seizures because these medications may worsen absence seizures.

Data Limitations

In the treatment of absence seizures there is often insufficient evidence for which of the available medications has the best combination of safety and efficacy for a particular patient. Nor is it easily known how long a medication must be continued before an off-medication trial should be conducted to determine whether the patient has outgrown the absence seizures, as is often the case in children. To date there have been no published results of any large, double-blind, placebo-controlled studies comparing the efficacy and safety of these or any other medications for absence seizures. The studies that exist have been small and not produced clear conclusions.

Myoclonus

Myoclonus is a brief, involuntary twitching of a muscle or a group of muscles. It describes a medical sign and, generally, is not a diagnosis of a disease. These myoclonic twitches, jerks, or seizures are usually caused by sudden muscle contractions (*positive myoclonus*) or brief lapses of contraction (*negative myoclonus*). The most common circumstance under which they occur is while falling asleep (hypnic jerk). Myoclonic jerks occur in healthy persons and are experienced occasionally by everyone. However, when they appear with more persistence and become more widespread they can be a sign of various neurological disorders. Hiccups are a kind of myoclonic jerk specifically affecting the diaphragm. When a spasm is caused by another person it is known as a *provoked spasm*. Shuddering attacks in babies fall in this category.

Myoclonic jerks may occur alone or in sequence, in a pattern or without pattern. They may occur infrequently or many times each minute. Most often, myoclonus is one of several signs in a wide variety of nervous system disorders such as multiple sclerosis, Parkinson's disease, Dystonia, Alzheimer's disease, Gaucher's disease, subacute sclerosing panencephalitis, Creutzfeldt–Jakob disease (CJD), serotonin toxicity, some cases of Huntington's disease, some forms of epilepsy, and occasionally in intracranial hypotension. Some researchers indicate that jerks persistently may even cause early tremors.

In almost all instances in which myoclonus is caused by central nervous system disease it is preceded by other symptoms; for instance, in CJD it is generally a late-stage clinical feature that appears after the patient has already started to exhibit gross neurological deficits.

Anatomically, myoclonus may originate from lesions of the cortex, subcortex or spinal cord. The presence of myoclonus above the foramen magnum effectively excludes spinal myoclonus; further localisation relies on further investigation with electromyography (EMG) and electroencephalography (EEG).

Symptoms

Myoclonic seizure can be described as "jumps" or "jolts" experienced in a single extremity or even the entire body. The feeling experienced by the individual is described as uncontrollable jolts common to receiving a mild electric shock. The sudden jerks and twitching of the body can often be so severe that it can cause a small child to fall.

A myoclonic seizure (*myo* "muscle", *clonic* "jerk") is a sudden involuntary contraction of muscle groups. The muscle jerks consist of symmetric, mostly generalized jerks, localized in the arms and in the shoulders and also simultaneously with a head nod; both the arms may fling out together and simultaneously a head nod may occur. Symptoms have some variability amongst subjects. Sometimes the entire body may jerk, just like a startle response. As is the case with all generalised seizures, the patient is not conscious during the event but the seizure is so brief that the person appears to remain fully conscious.

In reflex epilepsies, myoclonic seizures can be brought on by flashing lights or other environmental triggers.

Familiar examples of normal myoclonus include hiccups and hypnic jerks that some people experience while drifting off to sleep. Severe cases of pathologic myoclonus can distort movement and severely limit a person's ability to sleep, eat, talk, and walk. Myoclonic jerks commonly occur in individuals with epilepsy.

Types

The most common types of myoclonus include action, cortical reflex, essential, palatal, those seen in the progressive myoclonus epilepsies, reticular reflex, sleep and stimulus-sensitive.

Epilepsy Forms

- Cortical reflex myoclonus is thought to be a type of epilepsy that originates in the cerebral cortex – the outer layer, or «gray matter,» of the brain, responsible for much of the information processing that takes place in the brain. In this type of myoclonus, jerks usually involve only a few muscles in one part of the body, but jerks involving many muscles may occur. Cortical reflex myoclonus can be intensified when patients attempt to move in a certain way or perceive a particular sensation.
- Essential myoclonus occurs in the absence of epilepsy or other apparent abnormalities in the brain or nerves. It can occur randomly in people with no family history, or among members of the same family, indicating that it sometimes may be an inherited disorder. Essential myoclonus tends to be stable without increasing in severity over time. Some scientists speculate that some forms of essential myoclonus may be a type of epilepsy with no known cause.
- Juvenile myoclonic epilepsy JME usually consists of jerking and muscle twitches of the upper extremities. This may include the arms, shoulders, elbows, and are very rarely but not limited to the legs. JME is amongst the most common types of epilepsy and can affect one of every 14 people with the disease. These seizures typically occur shortly after waking up. Onset for JME can be seen around puberty for most patients. Administration of medications that also treat multiple seizure types is usually the most effective form of treatment.
- Lennox-Gastaut syndrome LGS or childhood epileptic encephalopathy is a rare epileptic disorder accounting for 1-4% of childhood epilepsies. The syndrome has much more severe symptoms ranging from multiple seizures daily, mental retardation, abnormal findings in electroencephalogram (EEG). Earlier age of seizure onset is correlated with higher risk of cognitive impairment.
- Progressive myoclonus epilepsy (PME) is a group of diseases characterized by myoclonus, epileptic seizures, tonic-clonic seizures, and other serious symptoms such as trouble walking or speaking. These rare disorders often get worse over time and sometimes are fatal. Studies have identified at least three forms of PME. Lafora disease is inherited as an autosomal recessive dis-

order, meaning that the disease occurs only when a child inherits two copies of a defective gene, one from each parent. Lafora disease is characterized by myoclonus, epileptic seizures, and dementia (progressive loss of memory and other intellectual functions). A second group of PME diseases belonging to the class of cerebral storage diseases usually involves myoclonus, visual problems, dementia, and dystonia (sustained muscle contractions that cause twisting movements or abnormal postures). Another group of PME disorders in the class of system degenerations often is accompanied by action myoclonus, seizures, and problems with balance and walking. Many of these PME diseases begin in childhood or adolescence. Treatment is not normally successful for any extended period of time.

- Reticular reflex myoclonus is thought to be a type of generalized epilepsy that originates in the brainstem, the part of the brain that connects to the spinal cord and controls vital functions such as breathing and heartbeat. Myoclonic jerks usually affect the whole body, with muscles on both sides of the body affected simultaneously. In some people, myoclonic jerks occur in only a part of the body, such as the legs, with all the muscles in that part being involved in each jerk. Reticular reflex myoclonus can be triggered by either a voluntary movement or an external stimulus.

Diaphragmatic Flutter

A very rare form includes the diaphragmatic flutter, the Belly Dancer's Syndrome, or Van Leeuwenhoek's disease. It was first described by Antony van Leeuwenhoek in 1723, who suffered from it. The condition characterizes spoken communication that sounds like a short-breathed hiccup. These muscle spasms can recur dozens of times per day. Rate of diaphragmatic contraction ranges between 35 and 480 contractions per minute, with the average rate found to be 150. Studies show that possible causes include disruptions within the central or peripheral nervous systems, anxiety, nutritional disorder, and certain pharmaceuticals. No single treatment has proven effective, though blocking or crushing of the phrenic nerve can provide instantaneous relief when pharmacologic treatment has proven ineffective.

Only about 50 people in the world have been diagnosed with diaphragmatic flutter. One case is Chaz Moore of Colorado Springs, Colorado, who was interviewed by CNN's Dr. Sanjay Gupta. The patient had tried several medications, of which only medical marijuana worked.

Other Forms

- Action myoclonus is characterized by muscular jerking triggered or intensified by voluntary movement or even the intention to move. It may be made worse by attempts at precise, coordinated movements. Action myoclonus is the most disabling form of myoclonus and can affect the arms, legs, face, and even the voice. It is often associated with tonic-clonic seizures and diffuse neuronal disease such as post-hypoxic encephalopathy, uremia, and the various forms of PME, although, in the case of focal cerebral damage, the disease may be restricted to one limb. This type of myoclonus often is caused by brain damage that results from a lack of oxygen and blood flow to the brain when breathing or heartbeat is temporarily stopped. Overexcitement of the sensorimotor cortex (Cortical Reflex Myoclonus) or reticular formation (Reticular Reflex Myoclonus) is also a cause of action myoclonus. Serotonin and GABA neurotransmitters are thought to cause this lack of inhibition, which is a possible explanation as to why improvements are made with the administration of serotonin precursors. Systems involved include the cerebellodentatorubral, pyramidal, extrapyramidal, optic, auditory, posterior columns and gracile and cuneate nuclei, spinocerebellar tracts, motor neurons of cranial nerves and anterior horns, and muscle fibers.

- Palatal myoclonus is a regular, rhythmic contraction of one or both sides of the rear of the roof of the mouth, called the soft palate. These contractions may be accompanied by myoclonus in other muscles, including those in the face, tongue, throat, and diaphragm. The contractions are very rapid, occurring as often as 150 times a minute, and may persist during sleep. The condition usually appears in adults and can last indefinitely. People with palatal myoclonus usually regard it as a minor problem; some complain of an occasional "clicking" sound, a noise made as the soft palate muscles contract.

- Middle ear myoclonus occurs in the muscles of the middle ear. These muscles may include the tensor tympani and stapedius muscles. It can involve the muscles surrounding the Eustachian tube, which include the tensor veli palatini, levator veli palatini, and salpingopharyngeus. Sufferers describe it as a thumping sound or sensation in the ear.

- Spinal myoclonus is myoclonus originating in the spinal cord, including segmental and propriospinal myoclonus. The latter is usually due to a thoracic generator producing truncal flexion jerk. It is often stimulus-induced with a delay due to the slow conducting propriospinal nerve fibers.

- Stimulus-sensitive myoclonus is triggered by a variety of external events, including noise, movement, and light. Surprise may increase the sensitivity of the patient.

- Sleep myoclonus occurs during the initial phases of sleep, especially at the moment of dropping off to sleep. Some forms appear to be stimulus-sensitive. Some people with sleep myoclonus are rarely troubled by it, or need treatment. If it is a symptom of a more complex and disturbing sleep disorders, such as restless legs syndrome, it may require medical treatment. Myoclonus can be associated with patients with Tourette syndrome.

Cause

Benign myoclonus can occur in healthy individuals and is most commonly caused by nothing other than arbitrary muscle contractions. Myoclonus may develop in response to infection, hyperosmolar hyperglycemic state, head or spinal cord injury, stroke, stress, brain tumors, kidney or liver failure, lipid storage disease, chemical or drug poisoning, as a side effect of certain drugs (such as tramadol, quinolones, benzodiazepine, gabapentin, sertraline, lamotrigine), or other disorders.

Benign myoclonic movements are commonly seen during the induction of general anesthesia with intravenous medications such as etomidate and propofol. These are postulated to result from decreased inhibitory signaling from cranial neurons. Prolonged oxygen deprivation to the brain, hypoxia, may result in posthypoxic myoclonus. People suffering from benign fasciculation syndrome can often experience myoclonic jerking of limbs, fingers and thumbs.

Myoclonus can occur by itself, but most often as one of several symptoms associated with a variety of nervous system disorders, including multiple sclerosis, Parkinson's disease, Alzheimer's disease, Opsoclonus Myoclonus, Creutzfeldt–Jakob disease, Lyme Disease and lupus. Myoclonic jerks commonly occur in persons with epilepsy, a disorder in which the electrical activity in the brain becomes disordered leading to seizures. It is also found in MERRF (Myoclonic Epilepsy with Ragged Red Fibers), a rare mitochondrial encephalomyopathy. Myoclonus can be a coexisting condition with Tourette syndrome.

Jerks of muscle groups, much of the body, or a series in rapid succession, which results in the person jerking bolt upright from a more relaxed sitting position is sometimes seen in ambulatory patients being treated with high doses of morphine, hydromorphine, and similar drugs, and is possibly a sign of high and/or rapidly increasing serum levels of these drugs. Myoclonic jerks caused by other opioids, such as tramadol and pethidine, may be less benign. Medications unrelated to opioids, such as anticholinergics, are known to cause myoclonic jerks.

Pathophysiology

Most myoclonus is caused by a disturbance of the central nervous system. Some are from peripheral nervous system injury. Studies suggest several locations in the brain are involved in myoclonus. One is in the brainstem, close to structures that are responsible for the startle response, an automatic reaction to an unexpected stimulus involving rapid muscle contraction.

The specific mechanisms underlying myoclonus are not yet fully understood. Scientists believe that some types of stimulus-sensitive myoclonus may involve overexcitability of the parts of the brain that control movement. These parts are interconnected in a series of feedback loops called motor pathways. These pathways facilitate and modulate communication between the brain and muscles. Key elements of this communication are chemicals known as neurotransmitters, which carry messages from one nerve cell, or neuron, to another. Neurotransmitters are released by neurons and attach themselves to receptors on parts of neighboring cells. Some neurotransmitters may make the receiving cell more sensitive, while others tend to make the receiving cell less sensitive. Laboratory studies suggest that an imbalance between these chemicals may underlie myoclonus.

Some researchers speculate that abnormalities or deficiencies in the receptors for certain neurotransmitters may contribute to some forms of myoclonus. Receptors that appear to be related to myoclonus include those for two important inhibitory neurotransmitters: serotonin, which constricts blood vessels and brings on sleep, and gamma-aminobutyric acid (GABA), which helps the brain maintain muscle control. Other receptors with links to myoclonus include those for benzodiazepines, drugs that induce sleep, and for glycine, an inhibitory neurotransmitter that is important for the control of motor and sensory functions in the spinal cord. More research is needed to determine how these receptor abnormalities cause or contribute to myoclonus.

Treatment

Concerning more serious afflictions, the complex origins of myoclonus may be treated with multiple drugs, which have a limited effect individually, but greater when combined with others that act on different brain pathways or mechanisms. Treatment is most effective when the underlying cause is known, and can be treated as such. Some drugs being studied in different combinations include clonazepam, sodium valproate, piracetam, and primidone. Hormonal therapy may improve responses to antimyoclonic drugs in some people.

Some studies have shown that doses of 5-hydroxytryptophan (5-HTP) leads to improvement in patients with some types of action myoclonus and PME. These differences in the effect of 5-HTP on patients with myoclonus have not yet been explained.

Many of the drugs used for myoclonus, such as barbiturates, phenytoin and primidone, are also used to treat epilepsy. Barbiturates slow down the central nervous system and cause tranquilizing or antiseizure effects. Phenytoin and primidone are effective antiepileptics drugs, although phenytoin can cause liver failure or have other harmful long-term effects in patients with PME. Sodium valproate is an alternative therapy for myoclonus and can be used either alone or in combination with clonazepam. Some people have adverse reactions to clonazepam and/or sodium valproate.

When patients are taking multiple medications, the discontinuation of drugs suspected of causing myoclonus and treatment of metabolic derangements may resolve some cases of myoclonus. When pharmacological treatment is indicated anticonvulsants are the main line of treatment. Paradoxical reactions to treatment are notable. Drugs which most people respond to may in other individuals worsen their symptoms. Sometimes this leads to the mistake of increasing the dose, rather than decreasing or stopping the drug. Treatment of myoclonus focuses on medications that may help reduce symptoms. Drugs used include sodium valproate, clonazepam, the anticonvulsant levetiracetam, and piracetam. Dosages of clonazepam usually are increased gradually until the patient improves or side effects become harmful. Drowsiness and loss of coordination are common side effects. The beneficial effects of clonazepam may diminish over time if the patient develops a tolerance to the drug.

In forms of myoclonus where only a single area is affected, and even in a few other various forms, Botox injections (OnabotulinumtoxinA) may be helpful. The chemical messenger responsible for triggering the involuntary muscle contractions is blocked by the Botulinum toxins of the Botox.

Surgery is also a viable option for treatment if the symptoms are caused by a tumor or lesion in the brain or spinal cord. Surgery may also correct symptoms in those where myoclonus affects parts of the face or ear. While DBS is still being studied for use with myoclonus, Deep Brain Stimulation has also been tried in those with this and other movement disorders.

Prognosis

The effects of myoclonus in an individual can vary depending on the form and the overall health of the individual. In severe cases, particularly those indicating an underlying disorder in the brain or nerves, movement can be extremely distorted and limit ability to normally function, such as in eating, talking, and walking. In these cases, treatment that is usually effective, such as clonazepam and sodium valproate, may instead cause adverse reaction to the drug, including increased tolerance and a greater need for increase in dosage. However, the prognosis for more simple forms of myoclonus in otherwise healthy individuals may be neutral, as the disease may cause few to no difficulties. Other times the disease starts simply, in one region of the body, and then spreads.

Generalised Tonic-clonic Seizure

Tonic–clonic seizures (formerly known as grand mal seizures) are a type of generalized seizure that affects the entire brain. Tonic–clonic seizures are the seizure type most commonly associated with epilepsy and seizures in general, though it is a misconception that they are the only type.

Tonic–clonic seizures can be induced deliberately in electroconvulsive therapy.

Pathophysiology

The vast majority of generalized seizures are idiopathic. However, some generalized seizures start as a smaller seizure such as a simple partial seizure or a complex partial seizure and then spread to both hemispheres of the brain. This is called a secondary generalization. Factors could include chemical and neurotransmitter imbalances and a genetically determined seizure threshold, both of which have been implicated. The seizure threshold can be altered by fatigue, malnutrition, lack of sleep or rest, hypertension, stress, diabetes, the presence of neon or xenon strobe-flashes, fluorescent lighting, rapid motion or flight, blood sugar imbalances, anxiety, antihistamines and other factors.

In the case of symptomatic epilepsy, it is often determined by MRI or other neuroimaging techniques that there is some degree of damage to a large number of neurons. The lesions (i.e., scar tissue) caused by the loss of these neurons can result in groups of neurons forming a seizire 'focus' area, episodically firing abnormally, creating a seizure if the focus is not abolished or suppressed via anti-convulsant drugs.

Phases

A tonic–clonic seizure comprises two phases, the *tonic* phase and the *clonic* phase.

Tonic phase

> The patient will quickly lose consciousness (though not all generalized tonic-clonic seizures involve a full loss of consciousness), and the skeletal muscles will suddenly tense, often causing the extremities to be pulled towards the body or rigidly pushed away from it, which will cause the patient to fall if standing or sitting. The tonic phase is usually the shortest part of the seizure, usually lasting only a few seconds. The patient may also express brief vocalizations like a loud moan upon entering the beginning seizure with the tonic stage, due to air forcefully expelled from the lungs.

Clonic phase

> The patient's muscles will start to contract and relax rapidly, causing convulsions. These may range from exaggerated twitches of the limbs to violent shaking or vibrating of the stiffened extremities. The patient may roll and stretch as the seizure spreads. The eyes typically roll back or close. The lips or extremities may turn slightly bluish (cyanosis) and incontinence is seen in some cases.

It used to be thought of as helpful to put a spoon or other item in the persons mouth as to stop them swallowing their tongue. It is known this is not helpful now however and in fact is a choking/ injury hazard.

Due to physical, mental and nervous exhaustion, postictal sleep with stertorous breathing invariably follows a tonic–clonic seizure. Confusion and total amnesia upon regaining consciousness is usually experienced and slowly wears off as the patient becomes gradually aware that a seizure occurred and remembers who and what he is and where he is. Occasionally the patient may vomit or burst into tears from the experienced mental trauma. An additional smaller seizure can occur several minutes after the main seizure, particularly if the patient's seizure threshold has been brought unusually low by known factors or combinations of such - for example severe hangovers, sleep deprivation, prolonged physical tiredness or caffeine.

Atonic Seizure

Atonic seizures (also called drop seizures, akinetic seizures or drop attacks), are a type of seizure that consist of a brief lapse in muscle tone that are caused by temporary alterations in brain function. The seizures are brief - usually less than fifteen seconds. They begin in childhood and may persist into adulthood. The seizure itself causes no injury, but the loss of muscle control can result in direct injury from falling. Electroencephalography can be used to confirm diagnosis. It is rare and can be indicative of Lennox-Gastaut syndrome.

Atonic seizures can occur while standing, walking or sitting, and are often noticeable by a head drop (the neck muscles relaxing) and injury may result from hitting the face or head. As with common epileptic occurrences, no first aid is needed post-seizure, except in the instances where falling injuries have occurred. In some cases, a person may become temporarily paralyzed in part of his or her body. This usually does not last longer than 3 minutes.

Treatment

There is no general treatment for patients with a seizure disorder. Each treatment plan is specifically tailored to the individual patient based on their diagnosis and symptoms. Treatment options may include medical therapy, nerve stimulation, dietary therapy, or surgery, as appropriate. Clinical trials may also be a valuable treatment alternative. Usually, anticonvulsants are given based on other symptoms and / or associated problems. Because the areas of the cerebellum which determine increases and decreases in muscular tonus are close together, people experiencing atonic seizures are most likely experiencing myoclonic ones too, at some point. This may play a role in therapy and diagnostic.

Status Epilepticus

Status epilepticus (SE) is a single epileptic seizure lasting more than five minutes or two or more seizures within a five-minute period without the person returning to normal between them. Previous definitions used a 30-minute time limit. The seizures can be of the tonic–clonic type, with a regular pattern of contraction and extension of the arms and legs, or of types that do not involve contractions, such as absence seizures or complex partial seizures. Status epilepticus is a life-threatening medical emergency particularly if treatment is delayed.

Status epilepticus may occur in those with a history of epilepsy as well as those with an underlying problem of the brain. These underlying brain problems may include trauma, infections, or strokes among others. Diagnosis often involves checking the blood sugar, imaging of the head, a number of blood tests, and an electroencephalogram. Psychogenic nonepileptic seizures may present similarly. Other conditions that may also appear to be SE include low blood sugar, movement disorders, meningitis, and delirium among others.

Benzodiazepines are the preferred initial treatment after which typically phenytoin is given. Possible benzodiazepines include intravenous lorazepam as well as intramuscular injections of midazolam. A number of other medications may be used if these are not effective such as valproic acid, phenobarbital, propofol, or ketamine. Intubation may be required to help maintain the person's airway. Between 10 and 30% of people who have status epilepticus die within 30 days. The underlying cause, the person's age, and the length of the seizure are important factors in the outcome. Status epilepticus occurs in up to 40 per 100,000 people per year. It makes up about 1% of people who visit the emergency department.

Signs and Symptoms

Status epilepticus can be divided into two categories: convulsive and nonconvulsive (NCSE).

Convulsive

Convulsive status epilepticus presents with a regular pattern of contraction and extension of the arms and legs.

Epilepsia partialis continua is a variant involving hour-, day-, or even week-long jerking. It is a consequence of vascular disease, tumors, or encephalitis, and is drug-resistant.

Generalized myoclonus is commonly seen in comatose people following CPR and is seen by some as an indication of catastrophic damage to the neocortex.

Refractory status epilepticus is defined as status epilepticus that continues despite treatment with benzodiazepines and one antiepileptic drug.

Super-refractory status epilepticus is defined as status epilepticus that continues or recurs 24 hours or more after the onset of anaesthetic therapy, including those cases where status epilepticus recurs on the reduction or withdrawal of anesthesia.

Nonconvulsive

Nonconvulsive status epilepticus is a relatively long duration change in a person's level of consciousness without large scale bending and extension of the limbs due to seizure activity. It is of two main types with either prolonged complex partial seizures or absence seizures. Up to a quarter of cases of SE are nonconvulsive.

In the case of complex partial status epilepticus, the seizure is confined to a small area of the brain, normally the temporal lobe. Absence status epilepticus is marked by a generalized seizure affecting the whole brain. An EEG is needed to differentiate between the two conditions. This results in episodes characterized by a long-lasting stupor, staring, and unresponsiveness.

Causes

Only 25% of people who experience seizures or status epilepticus have epilepsy. The following is a list of possible causes:

- Stroke
- Hemorrhage
- Intoxicants or adverse reactions to drugs
- Insufficient dosage or sudden withdrawal of a medication (especially anticonvulsants)
- Consumption of alcoholic beverages while on an anticonvulsant, or alcohol withdrawal
- Dieting or fasting while on an anticonvulsant
- Starting on a new medication that reduces the effectiveness of the anticonvulsant or changes drug metabolism, decreasing its half-life, leading to decreased blood concentrations
- Developing a resistance to an anticonvulsant already being used
- Gastroenteritis while on an anticonvulsant, where lower levels of anticonvulsant may exist in the bloodstream due to vomiting of gastric contents or reduced absorption due to mucosal edema
- Developing a new, unrelated condition in which seizures are coincidentally also a symptom, but are not controlled by an anticonvulsant already used
- Metabolic disturbances—such as affected kidney and liver
- Sleep deprivation of more than a short duration is often the cause of a (usually,

but not always, temporary) loss of seizure control; those whose seizures are inherently severe but otherwise controlled by medication can regress and have severe seizures or status epilepticus even if they are still taking their medication unless they regain their rest.

Diagnosis

Definitions vary, but currently it is defined as one continuous, unremitting seizure lasting longer than five minutes, or recurrent seizures without regaining consciousness between seizures for greater than five minutes. Previous definitions used a 30-minute time limit.

NCSE is believed to be under-diagnosed.

Treatments

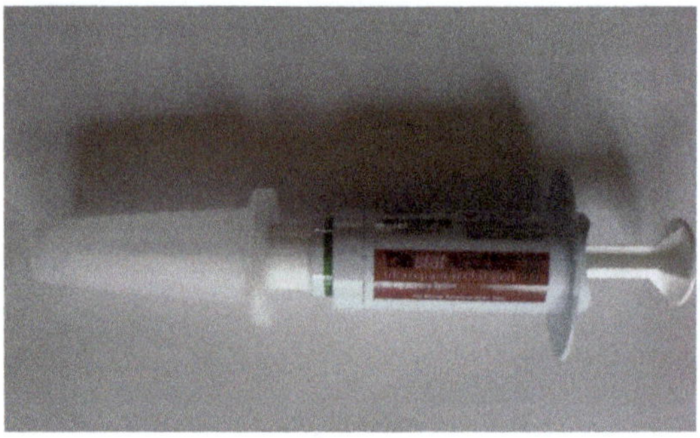

Diazepam that can be inserted rectally is often prescribed to caregivers of people with epilepsy. This enables treatment of multiple seizures prior to being able to seek medical care.

Benzodiazepines are the preferred initial treatment after which typically phenytoin is given. First aid guidelines for seizures state that, as a rule, an ambulance should be called for seizures lasting longer than five minutes (or sooner if this is the person's first seizure episode and no precipitating factors are known, or if SE happens to a person with epilepsy whose seizures were previously absent or well controlled for a considerable time period).

Benzodiazepines

When given intravenously, lorazepam appears to be superior to diazepam for stopping seizure activity. Intramuscular midazolam appears to be a reasonable option especially in those who are not in hospital.

The benzodiazepine of choice in North America for initial treatment is lorazepam due to its relatively long duration of action (2–8 hours) when injected, and its rapid onset of action, which is thought to be due to its high affinity for GABA receptors and to its low lipid solubility, which causes it to remain in the vascular compartment. If lorazepam is not available, or intravenous access is not possible, then diazepam should be given. In several countries outside North America, intravenous clonazepam is regarded as the drug of first choice. For instance a guideline from the Netherlands recommends clonazepam. Cited advantages of clonazepam include a longer duration of action than diazepam and a lower propensity for the development of acute tolerance than lorazepam. The use of clonazepam for this indication has not caught on in North America, as it is not available as an intravenous formulation there.

Particularly in children, another popular treatment choice is midazolam, given into the side of the mouth or the nose. Sometimes, the failure of lorazepam alone is considered to be enough to classify a case of SE as resistant to treatment.

Phenytoin and Fosphenytoin

Phenytoin was once another first-line therapy, although the prodrug fosphenytoin can be administered three times as fast and with far fewer injection site reactions. If these or any other hydantoin derivatives are used, then cardiac monitoring is a must if they are administered intravenously. Because the hydantoins take 15–30 minutes to work, a benzodiazepine or barbiturate is often coadministered. Because of diazepam's short duration of action, they were often administered together anyway.

Carbamazepine and Valproate

Valproate is available to be given intravenously, and may be used for status epilepticus. Carbamazepine is not available in an intravenous formulation, and does not play a role in status epilepticus.

Barbiturates

Before the benzodiazepines were invented, there were the barbiturates, which are still used today if benzodiazepines or the hydantoins are not an option. These are used to induce a barbituric coma. The barbiturate most commonly used for this is phenobarbital. Thiopental or pentobarbital may also be used for that purpose if the seizures have to be stopped immediately or if the person has already been compromised by the underlying illness or toxic/metabolic-induced seizures; however, in those situations, thiopental is the agent of choice.

Others

If this proves ineffective or if barbiturates cannot be used for some reason, then a general anesthetic such as propofol may be tried; sometimes it is used second after the failure of lorazepam. This also means putting the people on artificial ventilation. Propofol has been shown to be effective in suppressing the jerks seen in myoclonus status epilepticus.

Ketamine, an NMDA antagonist drug, can be used as a last resort for drug-resistant status epilepticus.

Lidocaine has been used in cases that do not improve with other more typical medications. One concern is that seizures often begin again 30 minutes after it is stopped. Additionally, it is not recommended in those with heart or liver problems.

Prognosis

Between 10 and 30% of people who have status epilepticus are dead within 30 days. The great majority of these people have an underlying brain condition causing their status seizure such as brain tumor, brain infection, brain trauma, or stroke. However, people with diagnosed epilepsy who have a status seizure also have an increased risk of death if their condition is not stabilized quickly, their medication and sleep regimen adapted and adhered to, and stress and other stimulant (seizure trigger) levels controlled. However, with optimal neurological care, adherence to the medication regimen, and a good prognosis (no other underlying uncontrolled brain or other organic disease), the person—even people who have been diagnosed with epilepsy—in otherwise good health can survive with minimal or no brain damage, and can decrease risk of death and even avoid future seizures.

Epidemiology

In the United States, about 40 cases of SE occur annually per 100,000 people. This includes about 10–20% of all first seizures.

Epilepsia Partialis Continua

Epilepsia partialis continua (also called Kojevnikov's or Kozhevnikov's epilepsia) is a rare type of brain disorder in which a patient experiences recurrent motor epileptic seizures that are focal (hands and face), and recur every few seconds or minutes for extended periods (days or years).

Presentation

During these seizures, there is repetitive focal myoclonus or Jacksonian march. After a seizure has subsided, Todd's phenomenon may be observed, which includes transient unilateral weakness.

Causes

There are numerous causes for this kind of seizure and they differ depending somewhat on the age at which the seizures begin. Epilepsy most often occurs at the extremes of life – in childhood or in very old age – but can develop at any time throughout one's life.

Although these seizures are usually due to large, acute brain lesions resulting from strokes in adults and focal cortical inflammatory processes in children (Rasmussen's encephalitis), possibly caused by chronic viral infections, edema, or autoimmune processes.

They are very medication and therapy-resistant, and the primary therapeutic goal is to stop secondary generalization. There are also many other reasons why these seizures occur. For example, they could be due to genetics, infections, or problems with brain development. Commonly the cause is unknown.

Genetic background determines such features as height, eye color, and potential to develop certain diseases like diabetes, but it also determines all the chemicals and structures that make up the brain, therefore playing a role in epilepsia partialis continua. The chemicals and structures that make up the brain have similarities across different people, but they vary in certain enzymes and receptors. These variations are not usually enough to cause a problem, but occasionally they do. For example, if a person has a mutation in a gene that creates the sodium channel (a part of the neuron required for firing) it makes it easier for neuronal firing to get out of control.

An infection of the brain (encephalitis) can also be a contributing factor. Although this sort of infection is uncommon it can be due to a virus, bacterium, or (very rarely) fungus. If a seizure happens during the infection itself, the person most likely doesn't have epilepsy, but has *"symptomatic seizures"* or seizures occurring because of a known injury to the brain. Once the infection is stopped the seizures will stop. Another more common infection is *"meningitis"*, infection of the membranes surrounding the brain. Since this infection does not directly involve the brain it might not appear as a possible cause of epilepsy, but has been shown that meningitis can cause epilepsy, which would give rise to the possibility of developing epilepsy partialis continua. These infections are most likely to result in epilepsy when they occur at an early age.

Problems with brain development can also be a factor. The brain undergoes a complicated process during development in which neurons are born and must travel to the surface of the brain. Here they wind up carefully placed in six distinct layers of the cerebral cortex. Throughout the brain the placement of these neurons are normally quite precise. If this system doesn't work exactly right, neurons can develop outside their appropriate areas. If this happens then the firing or circuitry of the brain is not right, and an abnormal, epileptic circuit can result.

Treatment

Identification of the underlying cause plays an important role in treatment. Brain abscesses or tumors can be—at least temporarily or partially, if not fully and permanently—surgically treated and chemotherapy and/or radiotherapy given to the patient. If seizures do continue, various anticonvulsant medication regimens that can be tolerated by the patient can be tested and if need be, administered, either orally, or in emergency conditions such as status epilepticus after tonic-clonic (grand mal) seizures, intravenously. If stroke or other similar, transient disorders occur (cerebrovascular accident, or transient ischemic attack, TIA), then neurological imaging of the affected lobes or hemispheres of the brain can be performed (CT, MRI, PET, etc.) and, if not absolutely contraindicated, antithrombolytic therapy might be given if it can be tolerated due to the seizures; if a hemorrhagic stroke has occurred and surgery can be performed to cauterize the vessel or otherwise stop the bleeding, it will be attempted if it can be done safely.

References

- Bradley, Walter G. (2012). "67". Bradley's neurology in clinical practice. (6th ed.). Philadelphia, PA: Elsevier/Saunders. ISBN 978-1437704341
- Walker, D. M.; Teach, S. J. (June 2006). "Update on the acute management of status epilepticus in children.". Curr Opin Pediatr. 18 (3): 239–44. PMID 16721142. doi:10.1097/01.mop.0000193306.55635.24
- Ahmad S, Beckett MW (2004). "Value of serum prolactin in the management of syncope". Emergency medicine journal : EMJ. 21 (2): e3. PMC 1726305. PMID 14988379. doi:10.1136/emj.2003.008870
- Steven C. Schachter, MD; Joseph I. Sirven, MD (July 2013). "Simple Partial Seizures". Epilepsy Foundation. Retrieved 31 August 2016
- Trinka, E; Höfler, J; Zerbs, A (September 2012). "Causes of status epilepticus.". Epilepsia. 53 Suppl 4: 127–38. PMID 22946730. doi:10.1111/j.1528-1167.2012.03622.x
- Nair, PP; Kalita, J.; Misra, U. K. (Jul–Sep 2011). "Status epilepticus: why, what, and how". Journal of Postgraduate Medicine. 57 (3): 242–52. PMID 21941070. doi:10.4103/0022-3859.81807
- "Epilepsy Action: Simple Partial Seizures". Epilepsy Action. British Epilepsy Association. 19 February 2008. Retrieved 2008-03-19
- Holmes, Thomas R. (2008). Handbook of epilepsy (4th ed.). Philadelphia: Lippincott Williams & Wilkins. p. 34. ISBN 978-0-7817-7397-3
- Dreifuss, FE (1983). "Treatment of the nonconvulsive epilepsies". Epilepsia. 24 Suppl 1: S45–54. PMID 6413201. doi:10.1111/j.1528-1157.1983.tb04642.x
- Wijdicks, Eelco F. M. (July 2002). "Propofol in myoclonus status epilepticus in comatose patients following cardiac resuscitation". Journal of Neurology Neurosurgery and Psychiatry. 73 (1): 94–5. PMC 1757284. PMID 12082068. doi:10.1136/jnnp.73.1.94
- Lava, Neil. "What is Juvenile Myonclonic Epilepsy". WebMD Medical Reference. Atlanta, Georgia: WebMD. Treatment of Juvenile Myoclonic Epilepsy. Retrieved 30 April 2015
- Daly, D. D. (1968). "Reflections on the Concept of Petit Mal". Epilepsia. 9 (3): 175–8. PMID 4975023. doi:10.1111/j.1528-1157.1968.tb04618.x
- Carlson, Neil (January 22, 2012). Physiology of Behavior. Neurological Disorders. 11th edition. Pearson. p. 550. ISBN 0-205-23939-0

5

Understanding Schizophrenia

Schizophrenia is a mental disorder which affects a person's ability to perceive reality. Symptoms include hearing voices, confusion, paranoia and alienation from the self. The chapter on schizophrenia offers an insightful focus, keeping in mind the complex subject matter.

Schizophrenia

Schizophrenia is a mental disorder characterized by abnormal social behavior and failure to understand what is real. Common symptoms include false beliefs, unclear or confused thinking, hearing voices that others do not hear, reduced social engagement and emotional expression, and a lack of motivation. People with schizophrenia often have additional mental health problems such as anxiety disorders, major depressive illness, or substance-use disorders. Symptoms typically come on gradually, begin in young adulthood, and last a long time.

The causes of schizophrenia include environmental and genetic factors. Possible environmental factors include being raised in a city, cannabis use, certain infections, parental age, and poor nutrition during pregnancy. Genetic factors include a variety of common and rare genetic variants. Diagnosis is based on observed behavior, the person's reported experiences, and reports of others familiar with the person. During diagnosis a person's culture must also be taken into account. As of 2013 there is no objective test. Schizophrenia does not imply a "split personality" or "multiple personality disorder" – conditions with which it is often confused in public perception.

The mainstay of treatment is antipsychotic medication, along with counselling, job training, and social rehabilitation. It is unclear whether typical or atypical antipsychotics are better. In those who do not improve with other antipsychotics clozapine may be tried. In more serious situations – where there is risk to self or others – involuntary hospitalization may be necessary, although hospital stays are now shorter and less frequent than they once were.

About 0.3–0.7% of people are affected by schizophrenia during their lifetimes. In 2013 there were an estimated 23.6 million cases globally. Males are more often affected than females. About 20% of people do well, and a few recover completely. Social problems, such as long-term unemployment, poverty, and homelessness are common. The average life expectancy of people with the disorder is ten to twenty-five years less than for the general population. This is the result of increased physical health problems and a higher suicide rate (about 5%). In 2015 an estimated 17,000 people worldwide died from behavior related to, or caused by, schizophrenia.

Signs and Symptoms

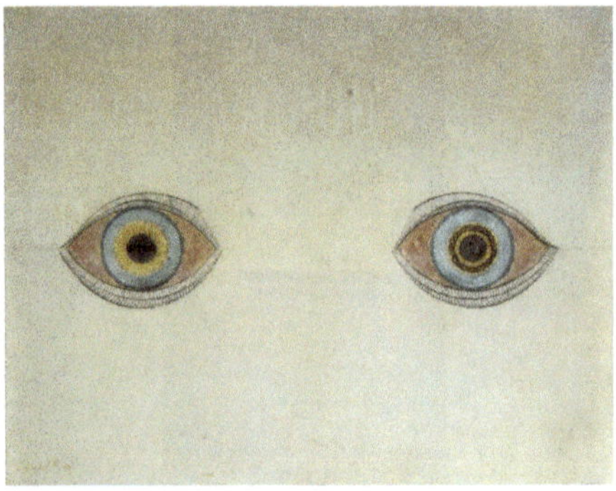

My Eyes at the Moment of the Apparitions by German artist August Natterer, who had schizophrenia

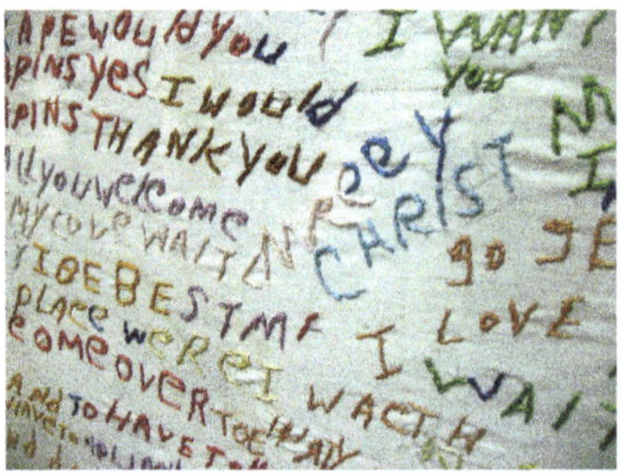

Cloth embroidered by a person diagnosed with schizophrenia

Individuals with schizophrenia may experience hallucinations (most reported are hearing voices), delusions (often bizarre or persecutory in nature), and disorganized thinking and speech. The last may range from loss of train of thought, to sentences only loosely connected in meaning, to speech that is not understandable known as word salad. Social withdrawal, sloppiness of dress and hygiene, and loss of motivation and judgment are all common in schizophrenia.

Distortions of self-experience such as feeling as if one's thoughts or feelings are not really one's own to believing thoughts are being inserted into one's mind, sometimes termed passivity phenomena, are also common. There is often an observable pattern of emotional difficulty, for example lack of responsiveness. Impairment in social cognition is associated with schizophrenia, as are symptoms of paranoia. Social isolation commonly occurs. Difficulties in working and long-term memory, attention, executive functioning, and speed of processing also commonly occur. In one uncommon subtype, the person may be largely mute, remain motionless in bizarre postures, or exhibit purposeless agitation, all signs of catatonia. People with schizophrenia often find facial emotion perception to be difficult. It is unclear if the phenomenon called "thought blocking", where a talking person suddenly becomes silent for a few seconds to minutes, occurs in schizophrenia.

About 30 to 50 percent of people with schizophrenia fail to accept that they have an illness or comply with their recommended treatment. Treatment may have some effect on insight.

People with schizophrenia may have a high rate of irritable bowel syndrome but they often do not mention it unless specifically asked. Psychogenic polydipsia, or excessive fluid intake in the absence of physiological reasons to drink, is relatively common in people with schizophrenia.

Positive and Negative

Schizophrenia is often described in terms of positive and negative (or deficit) symptoms. *Positive symptoms* are those that most individuals do not normally experience, but are present in people with schizophrenia. They can include delusions, disordered thoughts and speech, and tactile, auditory, visual, olfactory and gustatory hallucinations, typically regarded as manifestations of psychosis. Hallucinations are also typically related to the content of the delusional theme. Positive symptoms generally respond well to medication.

Negative symptoms are deficits of normal emotional responses or of other thought processes, and are less responsive to medication. They commonly include flat expressions or little emotion, poverty of speech, inability to experience pleasure, lack of desire to form relationships, and lack of motivation. Negative symptoms appear to contribute more to poor quality of life, functional ability, and the burden on others than positive symptoms do. People with greater negative symptoms often have a history of poor adjustment before the onset of illness, and response to medication is often limited.

Cognitive Dysfunction

Deficits in cognitive abilities are widely recognized as a core feature of schizophrenia. The extent of the cognitive deficits an individual experiences is a predictor of how functional an individual will be, the quality of occupational performance, and how successful the individual will be in maintaining treatment. The presence and degree of cognitive dysfunction in individuals with schizophrenia has been reported to be a better indicator of functionality than the presentation of positive or negative symptoms. The deficits impacting the cognitive function are found in a large number of areas: working memory, long-term memory, verbal declarative memory, semantic processing, episodic memory, attention, learning (particularly verbal learning). Deficits in verbal memory are the most pronounced in individuals with schizophrenia, and are not accounted for by deficit in attention. Verbal memory impairment has been linked to a decreased ability in individuals with schizophrenia to semantically encode (process information relating to meaning), which is cited as a cause for another known deficit in long-term memory. When given a list of words, healthy individuals remember positive words more frequently (known as the Pollyanna principle); however, individuals with schizophrenia tend to remember all words equally regardless of their connotations, suggesting that the experience of anhedonia impairs the semantic encoding of the words. These deficits have been found in individuals before the onset of the illness to some extent. First-degree family members of individuals with schizophrenia and other high-risk individuals also show a degree of deficit in cognitive abilities, and specifically in working memory. A review of the literature on cognitive deficits in individuals with schizophrenia shows that the deficits may be present in early adolescence, or as early as childhood. The deficits which an individual with schizophrenia presents tend to remain the same over time in most patients, or follow an identifiable course based upon environmental variables.

Although the evidence that cognitive deficits remain stable over time is reliable and abundant, much of the research in this domain focuses on methods to improve attention and working memory. Efforts to improve learning ability in individuals with schizophrenia using a high- versus low-reward condition and an instruction-absent or instruction-present condition revealed that increasing reward leads to poorer performance while providing instruction leads to improved performance, highlighting that some treatments may exist to increase cognitive performance. Training individuals with schizophrenia to alter their thinking, attention, and language behaviors by verbalizing tasks, engaging in cognitive rehearsal, giving self-instructions, giving coping statements to the self to handle failure, and providing self-reinforcement for success, significantly improves performance on recall tasks. This type of training, known as self-instructional (SI) training, produced benefits such as lower number of nonsense verbalizations and improved recall while distracted.

Onset

Late adolescence and early adulthood are peak periods for the onset of schizophrenia, critical years in a young adult's social and vocational development. In 40% of men and 23% of women diagnosed with schizophrenia, the condition manifested itself before the age of 19. To minimize the developmental disruption associated with schizophrenia, much work has recently been done to identify and treat the prodromal (pre-onset) phase of the illness, which has been detected up to 30 months before the onset of symptoms. Those who go on to develop schizophrenia may experience transient or self-limiting psychotic symptoms and the non-specific symptoms of social withdrawal, irritability, dysphoria, and clumsiness before the onset of the disease. Children who go on to develop schizophrenia may also demonstrate decreased intelligence, decreased motor development (reaching milestones such as walking slowly), isolated play preference, social anxiety, and poor school performance.

Causes

A combination of genetic and environmental factors play a role in the development of schizophrenia. People with a family history of schizophrenia who have a transient psychosis have a 20–40% chance of being diagnosed one year later.

Genetic

Estimates of heritability vary because of the difficulty in separating genetic and environmental influences; averages of 0.80 have been given. The greatest single risk factor for developing schizophrenia is having a first-degree relative with the disease (risk is 6.5%); more than 40% of monozygotic twins of those with schizophrenia are also affected. If one parent is affected the risk is about 13% and if both are affected the risk is nearly 50%.

Many genes are believed to be involved in schizophrenia, each of small effect and unknown transmission and expression. Many possible candidates have been proposed, including specific copy number variations, *NOTCH4*, and histone protein loci. A number of genome-wide associations such as zinc finger protein 804A have also been linked. There appears to be overlap in the genetics of schizophrenia and bipolar disorder. Evidence is emerging that the genetic architecture of schizophrenia involved both common and rare risk variation.

Assuming a hereditary basis, one question from evolutionary psychology is why genes that *increase* the likelihood of psychosis evolved, assuming the condition would have been maladaptive from an evolutionary point of view. One idea is that genes are involved in the evolution of language and human nature, but to date such ideas remain little more than hypothetical in nature.

Environment

Environmental factors associated with the development of schizophrenia include the living environment, drug use, and prenatal stressors.

Parenting style seems to have no major effect, although people with supportive parents do better than those with critical or hostile parents. Childhood trauma, death of a parent, and being bullied or abused increase the risk of psychosis. Living in an urban environment during childhood or as an adult has consistently been found to increase the risk of schizophrenia by a factor of two, even after taking into account drug use, ethnic group, and size of social group. Other factors that play an important role include social isolation and immigration related to social adversity, racial discrimination, family dysfunction, unemployment, and poor housing conditions.

It has been hypothesized that in some people, development of schizophrenia is related to intestinal tract dysfunction such as seen with non-celiac gluten sensitivity or abnormalities in the intestinal flora. A subgroup of persons with schizophrenia present an immune response to gluten different from that found in people with celiac, with elevated levels of certain serum biomarkers of gluten sensitivity such as anti-gliadin IgG or anti-gliadin IgA antibodies.

Substance use

About half of those with schizophrenia use drugs or alcohol excessively. Amphetamine, cocaine, and to a lesser extent alcohol, can result in a transient stimulant psychosis or alcohol-related psychosis that presents very similarly to schizophrenia. Although it is not generally believed to be a cause of the illness, people with schizophrenia use nicotine at much higher rates than the general population.

Alcohol abuse can occasionally cause the development of a chronic, substance-induced psychotic disorder via a kindling mechanism. Alcohol use is not associated with an earlier onset of psychosis.

Cannabis can be a contributory factor in schizophrenia, potentially causing the disease in those who are already at risk. The increased risk may require the presence of certain genes within an individual or may be related to preexisting psychopathology. Early exposure is strongly associated with an increased risk. The size of the increased risk is not clear, but appears to be in the range of two to three times greater for psychosis. Higher dosage and greater frequency of use are indicators of increased risk of chronic psychoses.

Other drugs may be used only as coping mechanisms by individuals who have schizophrenia, to deal with depression, anxiety, boredom, and loneliness.

Developmental Factors

Factors such as hypoxia and infection, or stress and malnutrition in the mother during fetal development, may result in a slight increase in the risk of schizophrenia later in life. People diagnosed with schizophrenia are more likely to have been born in winter or spring (at least in the northern hemisphere), which may be a result of increased rates of viral exposures in utero. The increased risk is about five to eight percent. Other infections during pregnancy or around the time of birth that may increase the risk include *Toxoplasma gondi* and *Chlamydia*.

Mechanisms

A number of attempts have been made to explain the link between altered brain function and schizophrenia. One of the most common is the dopamine hypothesis, which attributes psychosis to the mind's faulty interpretation of the misfiring of dopaminergic neurons.

Psychological

Many psychological mechanisms have been implicated in the development and maintenance of schizophrenia. Cognitive biases have been identified in those with the diagnosis or those at risk, especially when under stress or in confusing situations. Some cognitive features may reflect global neurocognitive deficits such as memory loss, while others may be related to particular issues and experiences.

Despite a demonstrated appearance of blunted affect, recent findings indicate that many individuals diagnosed with schizophrenia are emotionally responsive, particularly to stressful or negative stimuli, and that such sensitivity may cause vulnerability to symptoms or to the disorder. Some evidence suggests that the content of delusional beliefs and psychotic experiences can reflect emotional causes of the disorder, and that how a person interprets such experiences can influence symptomatology. The use of "safety behaviors" (acts such as gestures or the use of words in specific contexts) to avoid or neutralize imagined threats may actually contribute to the chronicity of delusions. Further evidence for the role of psychological mechanisms comes from the effects of psychotherapies on symptoms of schizophrenia.

Neurological

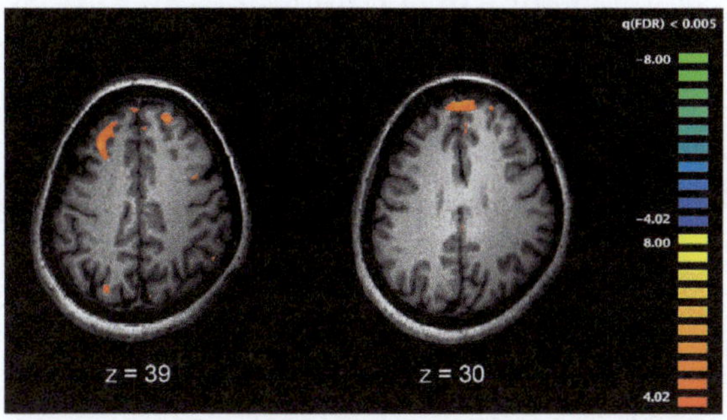

Functional magnetic resonance imaging (fMRI) showing two levels of the brain; areas in orange were more active in healthy controls than in medicated people with schizophrenia.

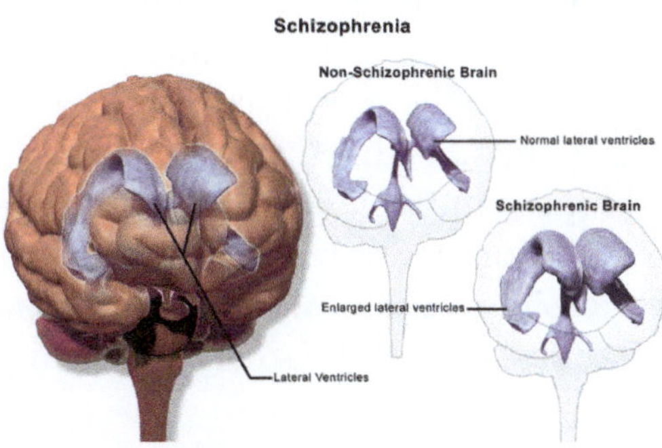

People with schizophrenia who are medication compliant have an association with enlarged lateral ventricles in the brain.

Schizophrenia is associated with subtle differences in brain structures, found in forty to fifty percent of cases, and in brain chemistry during acute psychotic states. Studies using neuropsychological tests and brain imaging technologies such as fMRI and PET to examine functional differences in brain activity have shown that differences seem to occur most commonly in the frontal lobes, hippocampus and temporal lobes. Reductions in brain volume, smaller than those found in Alzheimer's disease, have been reported in areas of the frontal cortex and temporal lobes. It is uncertain whether these volumetric changes are progressive or exist prior to the onset of the disease. These differences have been linked to the neurocognitive deficits often associated with schizophrenia. Because neural circuits are altered, it has alternatively been suggested that schizophrenia could be thought of as a neurodevelopmental disorder with psychosis occurring as a possibly preventable late stage. There has been debate on whether treatment with antipsychotics can itself cause reduction of brain volume.

Particular attention has been paid to the function of dopamine in the mesolimbic pathway of the brain. This focus largely resulted from the accidental finding that phenothiazine drugs, which block dopamine function, could reduce psychotic symptoms. It is also supported by the fact that amphetamines, which trigger the release of dopamine, may exacerbate the psychotic symptoms in schizophrenia. The influential dopamine hypothesis of schizophrenia proposed that excessive activation of D_2 receptors was the cause of (the positive symptoms of) schizophrenia. Although postulated for about 20 years based on the D_2 blockade effect common to all antipsychotics, it was not until the mid-1990s that PET and SPET imaging studies provided supporting evidence. Since the 2000s, several PET studies have confirmed an altered synthesis capacity of dopamine in the nigrostriatal system demonstrating a dopaminergic dysregulation. The dopamine hypothesis is now thought to be simplistic, partly because newer antipsychotic medication (atypical antipsychotic medication) can be just as effective as older medication (typical antipsychotic medication), but also affects serotonin function and may have slightly less of a dopamine blocking effect.

Interest has also focused on the neurotransmitter glutamate and the reduced function of the NMDA glutamate receptor in schizophrenia, largely because of the abnormally low levels of glutamate receptors found in the postmortem brains of those diagnosed with schizophrenia, and the discovery that glutamate-blocking drugs such as phencyclidine and ketamine can mimic the symptoms and cognitive problems associated with the condition. Reduced glutamate function is linked to poor performance on tests requiring frontal lobe and hippocampal function, and glutamate can affect dopamine function, both of which have been implicated in schizophrenia; this has suggested an important mediating (and possibly causal) role of glutamate pathways in the condition. But positive symptoms fail to respond to glutamatergic medication.

Diagnosis

Schizophrenia is diagnosed based on criteria in either the American Psychiatric Association's (APA) fifth edition of the *Diagnostic and Statistical Manual of Mental Disorders* (DSM 5), or the World Health Organization's International Statistical Classification of Diseases and Related Health Problems (ICD-10). These criteria use the self-reported experiences of the person and reported abnormalities in behavior, followed by a clinical assessment by a mental health professional. Symptoms associated with schizophrenia occur along a continuum in the population and must reach a certain severity and level of impairment, before a diagnosis is made. As of 2013 there is no objective test.

Criteria

In 2013, the American Psychiatric Association released the fifth edition of the DSM (DSM-5). To be diagnosed with schizophrenia, two diagnostic criteria have to be met over much of the time of a period of at least one month, with a significant impact on social or occupational functioning for at least six months. The person had to be suffering from delusions, hallucinations, or disorganized speech. A second symptom could be negative symptoms, or severely disorganized or catatonic behaviour. The definition of schizophrenia remained essentially the same as that specified by the 2000 version of DSM (DSM-IV-TR), but DSM-5 makes a number of changes.

- Subtype classifications – such as catatonic and paranoid schizophrenia – are removed. These were retained in previous revisions largely for reasons of tradition, but had subsequently proved to be of little worth.
- Catatonia is no longer so strongly associated with schizophrenia.
- In describing a person's schizophrenia, it is recommended that a better distinction be made between the current state of the condition and its historical progress, to achieve a clearer overall characterization.
- Special treatment of Schneider's first-rank symptoms is no longer recommended.
- Schizoaffective disorder is better defined to demarcate it more cleanly from schizophrenia.
- An assessment covering eight domains of psychopathology – such as whether hallucination or mania is experienced – is recommended to help clinical decision-making.

The ICD-10 criteria are typically used in European countries, while the DSM criteria are used in the United States and to varying degrees around the world, and are prevailing in research studies. The ICD-10 criteria put more emphasis on Schneiderian first-rank symptoms. In practice, agreement between the two systems is high. The current proposal for the ICD-11 criteria for schizophrenia recommends adding self-disorder as a symptom.

If signs of disturbance are present for more than a month but less than six months, the diagnosis of schizophreniform disorder is applied. Psychotic symptoms lasting less than a month may be diagnosed as brief psychotic disorder, and various conditions may be classed as psychotic disorder not otherwise specified, while schizoaffective disorder is diagnosed if symptoms of mood disorder are substantially present alongside psychotic symptoms. If the psychotic symptoms are the direct physiological result of a general medical condition or a substance, then the diagnosis is one of a psychosis secondary to that condition. Schizophrenia is not diagnosed if symptoms of pervasive developmental disorder are present unless prominent delusions or hallucinations are also present.

Subtypes

With the publication of DSM-5, the APA removed all sub-classifications of schizophrenia. The five sub-classifications included in DSM-IV-TR were:

- Paranoid type: Delusions or auditory hallucinations are present, but thought disorder, disorganized behavior, or affective flattening are not. Delusions are persecutory and/or grandiose, but in addition to these, other themes such as jealousy, religiosity, or somatization may also be present. (DSM code 295.3/ ICD code F20.0)
- Disorganized type: Named *hebephrenic schizophrenia* in the ICD. Where thought disorder and flat affect are present together. (DSM code 295.1/ICD code F20.1)
- Catatonic type: The subject may be almost immobile or exhibit agitated, purposeless movement. Symptoms can include catatonic stupor and waxy flexibility. (DSM code 295.2/ICD code F20.2)
- Undifferentiated type: Psychotic symptoms are present but the criteria for paranoid, disorganized, or catatonic types have not been met. (DSM code 295.9/ ICD code F20.3)
- Residual type: Where positive symptoms are present at a low intensity only. (DSM code 295.6/ICD code F20.5)

The ICD-10 defines two additional subtypes:

- Post-schizophrenic depression: A depressive episode arising in the aftermath of a schizophrenic illness where some low-level schizophrenic symptoms may still be present. (ICD code F20.4)
- Simple schizophrenia: Insidious and progressive development of prominent negative symptoms with no history of psychotic episodes. (ICD code F20.6)

Latent schizophrenia (F21.1), schizophrenic reaction (F21.2), pseudoneurotic schizophrenia (F21.3), pseudopsychopathic schizophrenia (F21.4), "symptom-depleted" schizophrenia (F21.5) are in the Russian version of the ICD-10. They are in the category of "schizotypal" disorder in section F21 of chapter V.

Differential Diagnosis

Psychotic symptoms may be present in several other mental disorders, including bipolar disorder, borderline personality disorder, drug intoxication, and drug-induced psychosis. Delusions ("non-bizarre") are also present in delusional disorder, and social withdrawal in social anxiety disorder, avoidant personality disorder and schizotypal personality disorder. Schizotypal personality disorder has symptoms that are similar but less severe than those of schizophrenia. Schizophrenia occurs along with obsessive-compulsive disorder (OCD) considerably more often than could be explained by chance, although it can be difficult to distinguish obsessions that occur in OCD from the delusions of schizophrenia. A few people withdrawing from benzodiazepines experience a severe withdrawal syndrome which may last a long time. It can resemble schizophrenia and be misdiagnosed as such.

A more general medical and neurological examination may be needed to rule out medical illnesses which may rarely produce psychotic schizophrenia-like symptoms, such as metabolic disturbance, systemic infection, syphilis, AIDS dementia complex, epilepsy, limbic encephalitis, and brain lesions. Stroke, multiple sclerosis, hyperthyroidism, hypothyroidism, and dementias such as Alzheimer's disease, Huntington's disease, frontotemporal dementia, and Lewy Body dementia may also be associated with schizophrenia-like psychotic symptoms. It may be necessary to rule out a delirium, which can be distinguished by visual hallucinations, acute onset and fluctuating level of consciousness, and indicates an underlying medical illness. Investigations are not generally repeated for relapse unless there is a specific *medical* indication or possible adverse effects from antipsychotic medication. In children hallucinations must be separated from typical childhood fantasies.

Prevention

Prevention of schizophrenia is difficult as there are no reliable markers for the later development of the disorder. There is tentative evidence for the effectiveness of early interventions to prevent schizophrenia. While there is some evidence that early intervention in those with a psychotic episode may improve short-term outcomes, there is little benefit from these measures after five years. Attempting to prevent schizophrenia in the prodrome phase is of uncertain benefit and therefore as of 2009 is not recommended. Cognitive behavioral therapy may reduce the risk of psychosis in those at high risk after a year and is recommended in this group, by the National Institute for Health and Care Excellence (NICE). Another preventative measure is to avoid drugs that have been associated with development of the disorder, including cannabis, cocaine, and amphetamines.

Management

The primary treatment of schizophrenia is antipsychotic medications, often in combination with psychological and social supports. Hospitalization may occur for severe episodes either voluntarily or (if mental health legislation allows it) involuntarily. Long-term hospitalization is uncommon since deinstitutionalization beginning in the 1950s, although it still occurs. Community support services including drop-in centers, visits by members of a community mental health team, supported employment and support groups are common. Some evidence indicates that regular exercise has a positive effect on the physical and mental health of those with schizophrenia.

Medication

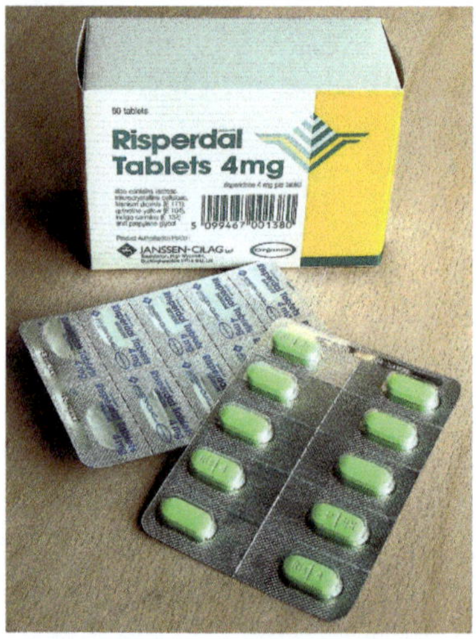

Risperidone (trade name Risperdal) is a common atypical antipsychotic medication.

The first-line psychiatric treatment for schizophrenia is antipsychotic medication, which can reduce the positive symptoms of psychosis in about 7 to 14 days. Antipsychotics, however, fail to significantly improve the negative symptoms and cognitive dysfunction. In those on antipsychotics, continued use decreases the risk of relapse. There is little evidence regarding effects from their use beyond two or three years. However use of anti-psychotics can lead to dopamine hypersensitivity increasing the risk of symptoms if antipsychotics are stopped.

The choice of which antipsychotic to use is based on benefits, risks, and costs. It is debatable whether, as a class, typical or atypical antipsychotics are better. Amisulpride, olanzapine, risperidone, and clozapine may be more effective but are associated with greater side effects. Typical antipsychotics have equal drop-out and symptom relapse rates to atypicals when used at low to moderate dosages. There is a good response in 40–50%, a partial response in 30–40%, and treatment resistance (failure of symptoms to respond satisfactorily after six weeks to two or three different antipsychotics) in 20% of people. Clozapine is an effective treatment for those who respond poorly to other drugs ("treatment-resistant" or "refractory" schizophrenia), but it has the potentially serious side effect of agranulocytosis (lowered white blood cell count) in less than 4% of people.

Most people on antipsychotics have side effects. People on typical antipsychotics tend to have a higher rate of extrapyramidal side effects, while some atypicals are associated with considerable weight gain, diabetes and risk of metabolic syndrome; this is most pronounced with olanzapine, while risperidone and quetiapine are also associated with weight gain. Risperidone has a similar rate of extrapyramidal symptoms to haloperidol. It remains unclear whether the newer antipsychotics reduce the chances of developing neuroleptic malignant syndrome or tardive dyskinesia, a rare but serious neurological disorder.

For people who are unwilling or unable to take medication regularly, long-acting depot preparations of antipsychotics may be used to achieve control. They reduce the risk of relapse to a greater degree than oral medications. When used in combination with psychosocial interventions, they may improve long-term adherence to treatment. The American Psychiatric Association suggests considering stopping antipsychotics in some people if there are no symptoms for more than a year.

Psychosocial

A number of psychosocial interventions may be useful in the treatment of schizophrenia including: family therapy, assertive community treatment, supported employment, cognitive remediation, skills training, token economic interventions, and psychosocial interventions for substance use and weight management. Family therapy or education, which addresses the whole family system of an individual, may reduce relapses and hospitalizations. Evidence for the effectiveness of cognitive-behavioral therapy (CBT) in either reducing symptoms or preventing relapse is minimal. Evidence for metacognitive training is mixed with one 2016 review finding benefit and another not. Art or drama therapy have not been well-researched. Music therapy has been shown to improve mental state and social functioning when paired with regular care.

Prognosis

Schizophrenia has great human and economic costs. It results in a decreased life expectancy by 10–25 years. This is primarily because of its association with obesity, poor diet, sedentary lifestyles, and smoking, with an increased rate of suicide playing a lesser role. Antipsychotic medications may also increase the risk. These differences in life expectancy increased between the 1970s and 1990s.

Schizophrenia is a major cause of disability, with active psychosis ranked as the third-most-disabling condition after quadriplegia and dementia and ahead of paraplegia and blindness. Approximately three-fourths of people with schizophrenia have ongoing disability with relapses and 16.7 million people globally are deemed to have moderate or severe disability from the condition. Some people do recover completely and others function well in society. Most people with schizophrenia live independently with community support. About 85% are unemployed. Some evidence suggests that paranoid schizophrenia may have a better prospect than other types of schizophrenia for independent living and occupational functioning. In people with a first episode of psychosis a good long-term outcome occurs in 42%, an intermediate outcome in 35% and a poor outcome in 27%. Outcomes for schizophrenia appear better in the developing than the developed world. These conclusions, however, have been questioned.

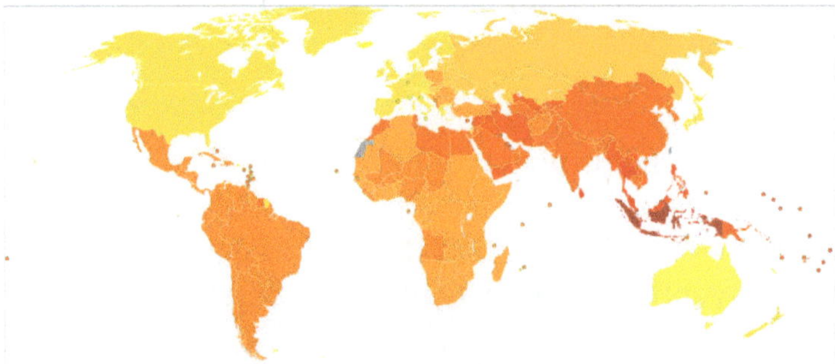

Disability-adjusted life years lost due to schizophrenia per 100,000 inhabitants in 2004.

no data	240–251
≤ 185	251–262
185–197	262–273
197–207	273–284
207–218	284–295
218–229	≥ 295
229–240	

There is a higher than average suicide rate associated with schizophrenia. This has been cited at 10%, but a more recent analysis revises the estimate to 4.9%, most often occurring in the period following onset or first hospital admission. Several times more (20 to 40%) attempt suicide at least once. There are a variety of risk factors, including male gender, depression, and a high intelligence quotient.

Schizophrenia and smoking have shown a strong association in studies worldwide. Use of cigarettes is especially high in individuals diagnosed with schizophrenia, with estimates ranging from 80 to 90% being regular smokers, as compared to 20% of the general population. Those who smoke tend to smoke heavily, and additionally smoke cigarettes with high nicotine content. Among people with schizophrenia use of cannabis is also common.

Epidemiology

Schizophrenia affects around 0.3–0.7% of people at some point in their life, or 24 million people worldwide as of 2011. It occurs 1.4 times more frequently in males than females and typically appears earlier in men—the peak ages of onset are 25 years for males and 27 years for females. Onset in childhood is much rarer, as is onset in middle or old age.

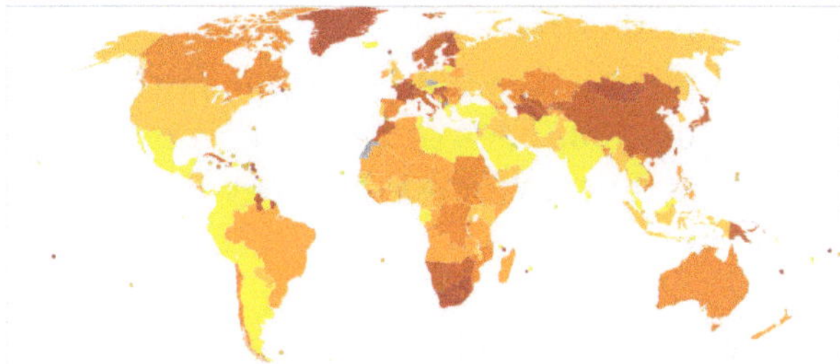
Deaths per million persons due to schizophrenia in 2012.

Despite the prior belief that schizophrenia occurs at similar rates worldwide, its frequency varies across the world, within countries, and at the local and neighborhood level. This variation has been estimated to be fivefold. It causes approximately one percent of worldwide disability adjusted life years and resulted in 20,000 deaths in 2010. The rate of schizophrenia varies up to threefold depending on how it is defined.

In 2000, the World Health Organization found the percentage of people affected and the number of new cases that develop each year is roughly similar around the world, with age-standardized prevalence per 100,000 ranging from 343 in Africa to 544 in Japan and Oceania for men, and from 378 in Africa to 527 in Southeastern Europe for women. About 1.1% of adults have schizophrenia in the United States.

History

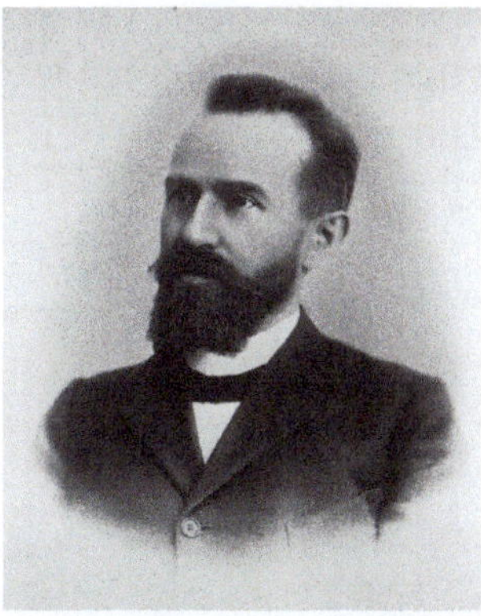
The term "schizophrenia" was coined by Eugen Bleuler.

In the early 20th century, the psychiatrist Kurt Schneider listed the forms of psychotic symptoms that he thought distinguished schizophrenia from other psychotic disorders. These are called *first-rank symptoms* or Schneider's first-rank symptoms. They include delusions of being controlled by an external force, the belief that thoughts are being inserted into or withdrawn from one's conscious mind, the belief that one's thoughts are being broadcast to other people, and hearing hallucinatory voices that comment on one's thoughts or actions or that have a conversation with other hallucinated voices. Although they have significantly contributed to the current diagnostic criteria, the specificity of first-rank symptoms has been questioned. A review of the diagnostic studies conducted between 1970 and 2005 found that they allow neither a reconfirmation nor a rejection of Schneider's claims, and suggested that first-rank symptoms should be de-emphasized in future revisions of diagnostic systems. The absence of first-rank symptoms should raise suspicion of a medical disorder, however.

The history of schizophrenia is complex and does not lend itself easily to a linear narrative. Accounts of a schizophrenia-like syndrome are thought to be rare in historical records before the 19th century, although reports of irrational, unintelligible, or uncontrolled behavior were common. A detailed case report in 1797 concerning James Tilly Matthews, and accounts by Philippe Pinel published in 1809, are often regarded as the earliest cases of the illness in the medical and psychiatric literature. The Latinized term *dementia praecox* was first used by German alienist Heinrich Schule in 1886 and then in 1891 by Arnold Pick in a case report of a psychotic disorder (hebephrenia). In 1893 Emil Kraepelin borrowed the term from Schule and Pick and in 1899 introduced a broad new distinction in the classification of mental disorders between *dementia praecox* and mood disorder (termed manic depression and including both unipolar and bipolar depression). Kraepelin believed that *dementia praecox* was probably caused by a long-term, smouldering systemic or "whole body" disease process that affected many organs and peripheral nerves in the body but which affected the brain after puberty in a final decisive cascade. His use of the term "praecox" distinguished it from other forms of dementia such as Alzheimer's disease which typically occur later in life. It is sometimes argued that the use of the term *démence précoce* in 1852 by the French physician Bénédict Morel constitutes the medical discovery of schizophrenia. However, this account ignores the fact that there is little to connect Morel's descriptive use of the term and the independent development of the *dementia praecox* disease concept at the end of the nineteenth century.

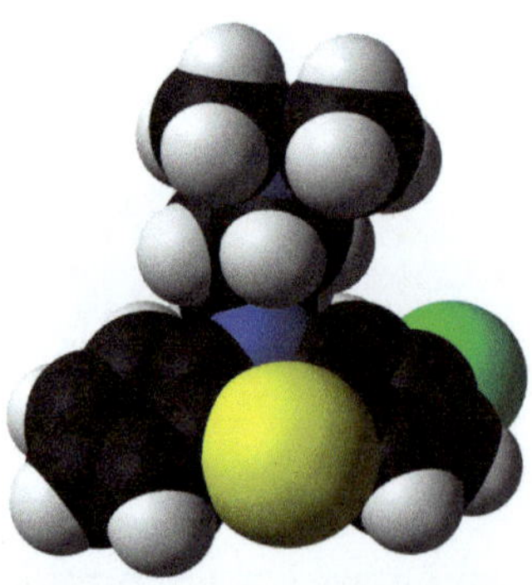

Molecule of chlorpromazine (trade name Thorazine), which revolutionized treatment of schizophrenia in the 1950s

The word *schizophrenia*—which translates roughly as "splitting of the mind" and comes from the Greek roots *schizein* and *phren* was coined by Eugen Bleuler in 1908 and was intended to describe the separation of function between personality, thinking, memory, and perception. American and British interpretations of Bleuler led to the claim that he described its main symptoms as four *A's*: flattened *affect*, *autism*, impaired *association* of ideas, and *ambivalence*. Bleuler realized that the illness was *not* a dementia, as some of his patients improved rather than deteriorated, and thus proposed the term schizophrenia instead. Treatment was revolutionized in the mid-1950s with the development and introduction of chlorpromazine.

In the early 1970s, the diagnostic criteria for schizophrenia were the subject of a number of controversies which eventually led to the operational criteria used today. It became clear after the 1971 US–UK Diagnostic Study that schizophrenia was diagnosed to a far greater extent in America than in Europe. This was partly due to looser diagnostic criteria in the US, which used the DSM-II manual, contrasting with Europe and its ICD-9. David Rosenhan's 1972 study, published in the journal *Science* under the title "On being sane in insane places", concluded that the diagnosis of schizophrenia in the US was often subjective and unreliable. These were some of the factors leading to the revision not only of the diagnosis of schizophrenia, but the revision of the whole DSM manual, resulting in the publication of the DSM-III in 1980.

The term schizophrenia is commonly misunderstood to mean that affected persons have a "split personality". Although some people diagnosed with schizophrenia may hear voices and may experience the voices as distinct personalities, schizophrenia does not involve a person changing among distinct, multiple personalities; the confusion arises in part due to the literal interpretation of Bleuler's term "schizophrenia" (Bleuler originally associated schizophrenia with dissociation, and included split personality in his category of schizophrenia). Dissociative identity disorder (having a "split personality") was also often misdiagnosed as schizophrenia based on the loose criteria in the DSM-II. The first known misuse of the term to mean "split personality" was in an article by the poet T. S. Eliot in 1933. Other scholars have traced earlier roots. Rather, the term means a "splitting of mental functions", reflecting the presentation of the illness.

Society and Culture

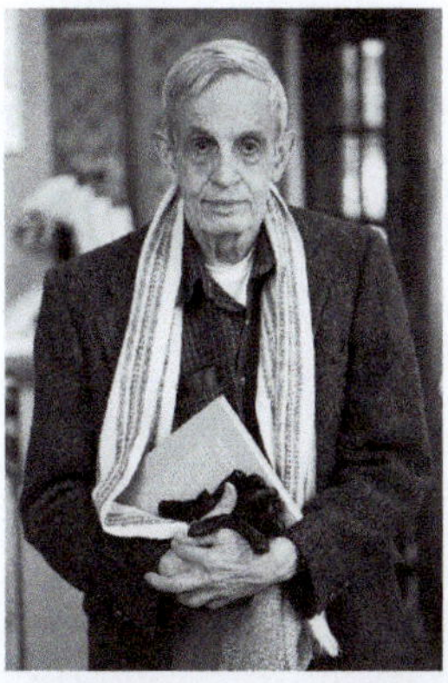

John Nash, an American mathematician and joint recipient of the 1994 Nobel Prize for Economics, who had schizophrenia. His life was the subject of the 2001 Academy Award-winning film *A Beautiful Mind*.

In 2002, the term for schizophrenia in Japan was changed from *seishin-bunretsu-byō* to reduce stigma. The new name was inspired by the biopsychosocial model; it increased the percentage of people who were informed of the diagnosis from 37 to 70% over three years. A similar change was made in South Korea in 2012. A professor of psychiatry, Jim van Os, has proposed changing the English term to "psychosis spectrum syndrome".

In the United States, the cost of schizophrenia–including direct costs (outpatient, inpatient, drugs, and long-term care) and non-health care costs (law enforcement, reduced workplace productivity, and unemployment)—was estimated to be $62.7 billion in 2002. The book and film *A Beautiful Mind* chronicles the life of John Forbes Nash, a Nobel Prize–winning mathematician who was diagnosed with schizophrenia.

Violence

Individuals with severe mental illness, including schizophrenia, are at a significantly greater risk of being *victims* of both violent and non-violent crime. Schizophrenia has been associated with a higher rate of violent acts, but most appear to be related to associated substance abuse. Rates of homicide linked to psychosis are similar to those linked to substance misuse, and parallel the overall rate in a region. What role schizophrenia has on violence independent of drug misuse is controversial, but certain aspects of individual histories or mental states may be factors. About 11% of people in prison for homicide have schizophrenia while 21% have mood disorders. Another study found about 8-10% of people with schizophrenia had committed a violent act in the past year compared to 2% of the general population.

Media coverage relating to violent acts by individuals with schizophrenia reinforces public perception of an association between schizophrenia and violence. In a large, representative sample from a 1999 study, 12.8% of Americans believed that individuals with schizophrenia were "very likely" to do something violent against others, and 48.1% said that they were "somewhat likely" to. Over 74% said that people with schizophrenia were either "not very able" or "not able at all" to make decisions concerning their treatment, and 70.2% said the same of money-management decisions. The perception of individuals with psychosis as violent has more than doubled in prevalence since the 1950s, according to one meta-analysis.

History of Schizophrenia

The word *schizophrenia* was coined by the Swiss psychiatrist and eugenicist Eugen Bleuler in 1908, and was intended to describe the separation of function between personality, thinking, memory, and perception. He formally introduced the term on 24 April 1908 in a lecture given at a psychiatric conference in Berlin and in a publication that same year. Bleuler later expanded his new disease concept into a monograph in 1911, which was finally translated into English in 1950.

The history of 'schizophrenia' is complex and not easy to characterize in a linear historical narrative, although attempts continue to be made. According to some, the disease has always existed only to be 'discovered' during the early 20th century. The plausibility of this claim depends upon the success of retrospectively diagnosing earlier cases of madness as 'schizophrenia'. According to others, 'schizophrenia' names a culturally determined clustering of mental symptoms. What is known for sure is that by the turn of the 20th century the old concept of insanity had become fragmented into 'diseases' (psychoses) such as paranoia, dementia praecox, manic-depressive insanity and epilepsy (Emil Kraepelin's classification). Dementia praecox was reconstituted as schizophrenia, paranoia was renamed as 'delusional disorder' and manic-depressive insanity as 'bipolar disorder' (epilepsy was transferred from psychiatry to neurology). It is important to emphasize that the 'mental symptoms' included under the concept schizophrenia are real enough, make people suffer, and will always need understanding and treatment. However, whether the historical construct currently called 'schizophrenia' is required to achieve this therapeutic goal remains contentious.

Diagnoses in Ancient Times

Accounts of a schizophrenia-like syndrome are thought to be rare in the historical record prior to the 19th century, although reports of irrational, unintelligible, or uncontrolled behavior were common. There has been an interpretation that brief notes in the Ancient Egyptian Ebers papyrus may imply schizophrenia, but other reviews have not suggested any connection. A review of ancient Greek and Roman literature indicated that although psychosis was described, there was no account of a condition meeting the criteria for schizophrenia.

Bizarre psychotic beliefs and behaviors similar to some of the symptoms of schizophrenia were reported in Arabic medical and psychological literature during the Middle Ages. In *The Canon of Medicine*, for example, Avicenna described a condition somewhat resembling the symptoms of schizophrenia which he called *Junun Mufrit* (severe madness), which he distinguished from other forms of madness (*Junun*) such as mania, rabies and manic depressive psychosis. However, no condition resembling schizophrenia was reported in Şerafeddin Sabuncuoğlu's *Imperial Surgery*, a major Ottoman medical textbook of the 15th century. Given limited historical evidence, schizophrenia (as prevalent as it is today) may be a modern phenomenon, or alternatively it may have been obscured in historical writings by related concepts such as melancholia or mania.

Influential Earlier Concepts

A detailed case 1809 report by John Haslam concerning James Tilly Matthews, and a separate account by Philippe Pinel also published in 1809, are often regarded as the earliest cases of schizophrenia in the medical and psychiatric literature. The Latinized term *dementia praecox* entered psychiatry in 1886 in a textbook by asylum physician Heinrich Schüle (1840-1916) of the Illenau asylum in Baden. He used the term to refer to hereditarily predisposed individuals who were "wrecked on the cliffs of puberty" and developed acute dementia, while others developed the chronic condition of hebephrenia. Emil Kraepelin had cited Schüle's 1886 textbook in the 1887 second edition of his own textbook, Psychiatrie, and hence was familiar with this term at least six years before he himself adopted it. It later appeared in 1891 in a case report by Arnold Pick which argued that hebephrenia should be regarded as a form of dementia praecox. Kraepelin first used the term in 1893. In 1899 Emil Kraepelin introduced a broad new distinction in the classification of mental disorders between *dementia praecox* and mood disorder (termed manic depression and including both unipolar and bipolar depression). Kraepelin believed that *dementia praecox* was caused by a lifelong, smoldering systemic or "whole body" process of a metabolic nature that would eventually affect the functioning of the brain in a final decisive cascade. Hence, he believed the entire body—all the organs, glands and peripheral nervous system—was implicated in the natural disease process. Although he used the term "dementia," Kraepelin seemed to use the term synonymously with "mental weakness," mental defect," and "mental deterioration," but distinguished it from other uses of the term dementia, such as in Alzheimer's disease, which typically occur later in life. In 1853 Bénédict Morel used the term *démence précoce* (precocious or early dementia) to describe a group of young patients who were suffering from "stupor". It is sometimes argued that this first use of the term signals the medical discovery of schizophrenia. However, Morel employed the phrase in a purely descriptive sense and he did not intend to delineate a new diagnostic category. Moreover, his traditional conception of dementia differed significantly from that employed in the latter half of the nineteenth-century. Finally, there is no evidence that Morel's *démence précoce* had any influence on the later development of the *dementia praecox* concept by either Arnold Pick or Emil Kraepelin.

Kraepelin's classification slowly gained acceptance. There were objections to the use of the term "dementia" despite cases of recovery, and some defence of diagnoses it replaced such as adolescent insanity. The concept of adolescent insanity or developmental insanity had been advanced by Scottish psychiatrist Sir Thomas Clouston in 1873, describing a psychotic condition which generally afflicted those aged 18–24 years, particularly males, and in 30% of cases proceeded to 'a secondary dementia'.

Coinage in 1908

The word *schizophrenia*—which translates roughly as "splitting of the mind" and comes from the Greek roots—was coined by Eugen Bleuler in 1908 and was intended to describe the separation of function between personality, thinking, memory, and perception. Bleuler described the main symptoms as 4 *A's*: flattened *Affect*, *Autism*, impaired *Association* of ideas and *Ambivalence*. Bleuler realized that the illness was not a dementia as some of his patients improved rather than deteriorated and hence proposed the term schizophrenia instead. However, many at the time did not accept that splitting or dissociation was an appropriate description, and the term would later have more significance as a source of confusion and social stigma than scientific meaning.

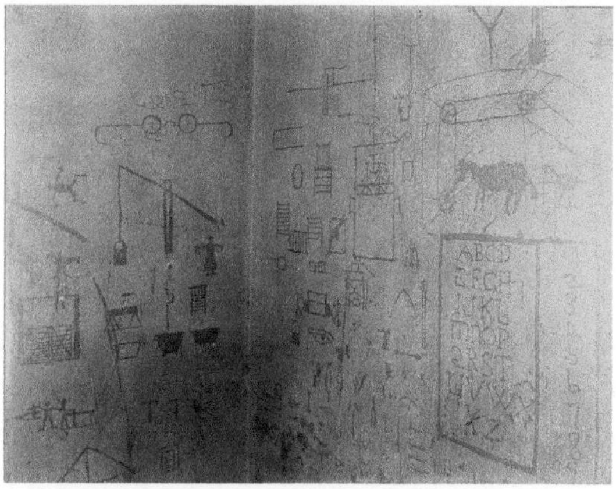

Scratch-drawings on the wall in St. Elizabeths Hospital made by a prisoner with "a disturbed case of dementia praecox".

In popular culture, the term *schizophrenia* is often thought to mean that affected persons have a "split personality". But for contemporary psychiatry, schizophrenia does not involve a person changing among distinct multiple personalities. The stigmatising confusion arises in part due to Bleuler's own use of the term *schizophrenia*, which for many signalled a split mind, and his documenting of a number of cases with split personalities within his classic 1911 description of schizophrenia. The earliest known use of the term to mean "split personality" was by Psychologist G. Stanley Hall in 1916. And many early 20th century psychiatrists and psychologists can also be found using the term in this sense (indeed some reference Jekyll and Hyde) before a later rejection of this usage took place.

In the early 20th century, the psychiatrist Kurt Schneider listed the forms of psychotic symptoms that he thought distinguished schizophrenia from other psychotic disorders. These are called *first-rank symptoms* or Schneider's first-rank symptoms. They include delusions of being controlled by an external force; the belief that thoughts are being inserted into or withdrawn from one's conscious mind; the belief that one's thoughts are being broadcast to other people; and hearing hallucinatory voices that comment on one's thoughts or actions or that have a conversation with other hallucinated voices. Although they have significantly contributed to the current diagnostic criteria, the specificity of first-rank symptoms has been questioned. A review of the diagnostic studies conducted between 1970 and 2005 found that they allow neither a reconfirmation nor a rejection of Schneider's claims, and suggested that first-rank symptoms should be de-emphasized in future revisions of diagnostic systems.

In the first half of the 20th century schizophrenia was considered to be a hereditary defect, and sufferers were subject to eugenics in many countries. Hundreds of thousands were sterilized, with or without consent—the majority in Nazi Germany, the United

States, and Scandinavian countries. Along with other people labeled "mentally unfit", many diagnosed with schizophrenia were murdered in the Nazi "Action T4" program.

Anti-psychiatry

Anti-psychiatry refers to a diverse collection of thoughts and thinkers that challenge the medical concept of schizophrenia. Anti-psychiatry emphasizes the social context of mental illness and re-frames the diagnosis of schizophrenia as a labeling of deviance. Anti-psychiatry represented dissension of psychiatrists themselves about the understanding of schizophrenia in their own field. Prominent psychiatrists in this movement include R. D. Laing, David Cooper. Related criticisms of psychiatry were launched by philosophers such as Michel Foucault, Jacques Lacan, Gilles Deleuze, Thomas Szasz, and Félix Guattari.

Anti-psychiatrists agree that 'schizophrenia' represents a problem, and that many human beings have problems living in modern society. But they protest the notion that schizophrenia is a disease, and that people who suffer from it are sick. Instead, they often suggest that schizophrenics appear crazy because they are intelligent and sensitive beings confronted with a mad world. The sane patient can choose to go Against medical advice, but the insane usually can not. Anti-psychiatry often describes the institutional world as itself pathological and insane because of the way it subordinates human beings to bureaucracy, protocol, and labels.

Controversies Over Validity in the 1970s

In 1970 psychiatrists Robins and Guze introduced new criteria for deciding on the validity of a diagnostic category and proposed that cases of schizophrenia where people recovered well were not really schizophrenia but a separate condition.

In the early 1970s, the diagnostic criteria for schizophrenia was the subject of a number of controversies which eventually led to the operational criteria used today. It became clear after the 1971 US-UK Diagnostic Study that schizophrenia was diagnosed to a far greater extent in America than in Europe. This was partly due to looser diagnostic criteria in the US, which used the DSM-II manual, contrasting with Europe and its ICD-9. David Rosenhan's 1972 study, published in the journal *Science* under the title *On being sane in insane places*, concluded that the diagnosis of schizophrenia in the US was often subjective and unreliable.

Politicization in the Soviet Union

In the Soviet Union the diagnosis of schizophrenia has also been used for political purposes. The prominent Soviet psychiatrist Andrei Snezhnevsky created and promoted an additional sub-classification of sluggishly progressing schizophrenia. This diagnosis was used to discredit and expeditiously imprison political dissidents while dispensing with a potentially embarrassing trial. The practice was exposed to Westerners by a number of Soviet dissidents, and in 1977 the World Psychiatric Association condemned the Soviet practice at the Sixth World Congress of Psychiatry. Rather than defending his claim that a latent form of schizophrenia caused dissidents to oppose the regime, Snezhnevsky broke all contact with the West in 1980 by resigning his honorary positions abroad.

DSM III (1980)

The 1970s controversies lead to the revision not only of the diagnosis of schizophrenia, but the revision of the whole DSM manual, resulting in the publication of the DSM-III in 1980. The revision was based on Feighner Criteria and Research Diagnostic Criteria that had in turn developed from Robins' and Guze's criteria, and which were intended to make diagnosis more reliable (consistent). Since the 1970s more than 40 diagnostic criteria for schizophrenia have been proposed and evaluated.

Evolution of Schizophrenia

The evolution of schizophrenia refers to the theory of natural selection working in favor of selecting traits that are characteristic of the disorder. Positive symptoms are features that are not present in healthy individuals but appear as a result of the disease process. These include visual and/or auditory hallucinations, delusions, paranoia, and major thought disorders. Negative symptoms refer to features that are normally present but are reduced or absent as a result of the disease process, including social withdrawal, apathy, anhedonia, alogia, and behavioral perseveration. Cognitive symptoms of schizophrenia involve disturbances in executive functions, working memory impairment, and inability to sustain attention. Given the high numbers of individuals diagnosed with schizophrenia (nearly 1% of modern-day populations), it is unlikely that the disorder has arisen solely from random mutations. Instead it is believed that despite its maladaptive nature, schizophrenia has been either selected for throughout the years or exists as an unwanted byproduct which accompanies desired genes.

Hypotheses

Social Brain Hypothesis

A social brain refers to the higher cognitive and affective systems of the brain, evolving as a result of social selection and serving as the basis for social interaction; it is the basis of the complexity of social interactions of which humans are capable. Mechanisms comprising the social brain include emotional processing, theory of mind, self-referencing, prospection and working memory. Patients display defects in various regions of the social brain, such as an inability to grasp social goals, which serves as an indication of a defect in theory of mind. As schizophrenia is foremost a disorder of the consciousness, it has been suggested that schizophrenia exists as an unwanted byproduct of the evolution of the prefrontal cortex and other brain regions constituting the social brain. Under increasingly selective pressure induced by increasingly complex social living, the regions of the brain have grown as a means of accommodation and in turn have given rise to vulnerable neural systems, allowing for psychoses such as schizophrenia to appear.

Social Advantage Hypothesis

This hypothesis refers to the worship of psychics and seers in the times of early civilization; the hallucinatory behavior and delusions brought by schizophrenia may have been highly regaled and allowed the individual to be conferred the title of saint or prophet, raising him on the social spectrum and allowing for social selection to act on the behalf of the disorder. This hypothesis lacks evidence and has not aided in explaining the continued persistence of schizophrenia in modern-day society where this idea of saints and prophets has no role.

Physiological Advantage Hypothesis

This hypothesis maintains that schizophrenics possess a physiological advantage in the form of disease or infection resistance, a theory that has found basis in diseases such as sickle-cell anemia. In one particular study, NAD, an energy carrier found in animals and yeast, is found to be capable of diminishing infectivity of tuberculosis when present in large quantities; this is done by repressing gene expression. However, *M. tuberculosis* bacterium has been shown to be capable of acting as a drain on NAD supply. Studies in kynurenine pathway activation reveal that *M. tuberculosis* infection of the pathway causes niacin receptors in the pathway to indicate high levels of niacin, a precursor to NAD that makes *de novo* synthesis of NAD from tryptophan unnecessary. This change creates the illusion that NAD levels are adequate and that tryptophan conversion is unnecessary. Coevolution with *M. tuberculosis* has resulted in an attempt to overcome this illusion in a variety of manners, including the up-regulation of niacin receptors and up-regulation of *de novo* synthesis of NAD from tryptophan via the kynurenine pathway. An enzyme implicated in the initiation of the kynurenine pathway, tryptophan 2,3-dioxygenase (TDO2) is found to activate during niacin-deficient conditions and is also found to be in increased levels in schizophrenic brains. In the postmortem brain tissue of schizophrenics, the protein for the high affinity niacin receptor was significantly decreased and, as a result, would allow for the up-regulation of mRNA transcript for the niacin receptor.

Shamanistic Hypothesis

This hypothesis purports that schizophrenia is a vestigial behaviour that was once adaptive to hunting and gathering tribes. Psychosis prompts shamans to communicate with the imaginary spirit world, which results in the formation of religious myths. The shamanistic theory posits that the universal presence of shamanism in all hunting and gathering societies is likely due to heritable factors - the same heritable factors that support the worldwide distribution of schizophrenia. One modern version of the theory has invoked the evolutionary mechanism of group selection in order to explain the apparent genetic-based task specialization of shamanism.

Immune System Hypothesis

Perinatal exposure

It has been suggested that acute neuroinflammation during early fetal development may contribute to schizophrenia pathogenesis. The risk of schizophrenia is higher among those who experienced prenatal maternal viral infections like influenza, rubella, measles, and polio as well as bacterial or reproductive infections.The brain is highly sensitive to environmental insults during early development. Factors common to the immune response to a variety of pathogens are mediators in linking the commonalities between prenatal/ perinatal infection and neurodevelopmental disorders. One hypothesis suggests that enhanced expression of proinflammatory cytokines and other mediators of inflammation in the maternal, fetal, and neonatal compartments may interfere with brain development, thereby increasing the risk for long-term brain dysfunction later in life.

Increased Pro-inflammatory Cytokines

Another hypothesis seeking to explain why schizophrenia occurs aim at understanding the activation of the immune system. The activation of the inflammatory response system mediated by cytokines may play a key role in the pathogenesis of schizophrenia. Evidence suggests that serum levels of IL-2, IL-6, IL-8, and TNF-α are significantly elevated in patients with chronic treatment-resistant schizophrenia. Nuclear factor-kappa B regulates the expression of cytokines and an increase in NF-κB levels leads to an increase in proinflammatory cytokine levels

Brain-derived Neurotrophic Factor

Individuals with schizophrenia have lower levels of brain-derived neurotrophic factor or BDNF. BDNF is responsible for promoting the proliferation, regeneration, and survival of neurons. It is also important for the regulation of cognitive function, something individuals with schizophrenia have trouble doing. Lower BDNF expression is associated with increased IL-6 expression, and increased cortisol levels. The more pro-inflammatory cytokines in circulation, the more the BDNF production decreases. This implies that an excess amount of pro-inflammatory cytokines negatively affects BDNF production. This, in turn, affects the presence and severity of psychosis in individuals with schizophrenia.

Self-domestication Hypothesis

The theory of self-domestication asserts that during the late Pleistocene period, archaic humans split from their hominid ancestors and underwent behavioral changes that led to a reduction of aggression and an increase in “tameness”. As a result of this transformation, changes to humans’ biological, morphological, physiological, and genetic development occurred; leading to anatomical changes in size, craniofacial structure, and brain structural differences, as well as changes in behavior related reduced levels of stress hormones and delayed maturation of the adrenal glands. The self-domestication hypothesis for evolution of schizophrenia observes the importance our self-domesticated evolution, with emphasis on its contribution to the altered genetic development of the neural crest and our relaxed our social cultural niche. Adaptations related these domesticated changes favored the emergence of complex cognitive abilities, including advanced linguistic cognition. The self-domestication hypothesis suggests that schizophrenia results from hypofunction of the neural crest development, triggered by the selection for domesticated “tameness”, and emphasize the domestic characteristics that make up the clinical phenotype of schizophrenia. Deficits related to language production and processing are prevalent in both positive and negative symptoms of schizophrenia. In addition, schizophrenic patients often demonstrate more marked domesticated traits at the morphological, physiological, and behavioral levels; including craniofacial abnormalities, desensitized cortical response to stress, and disorganized speech. A study published in 2017 targeted various candidate genes (*FOXD3, RET, SOX9, SOX10, GDNF*) with overlapping function in relation to schizophrenia, domestication, and neural crest development, and found the largest number of brain area expressions include to be in the frontal cortex, associate striatum nucleus, and hippocampus. Although the results do not reflect the molecular events that occurred during early neural development or evolution, they provide insight into the molecular network that underlies the impaired cognitive and social scenarios that act in the schizophrenic brain, and further suggest that self-domestication, language processing, and schizophrenia have an intimately intertwined relationship.

Extended Maturation Time Hypothesis

This hypothesis synthesizes two previous hypotheses for the evolution of schizophrenia involving humans’ development of functional brain asymmetry in the neocortex (Crow’s theory) and improvement of fatty acid metabolism (myelin production), while adding a third dynamic of mechanistic cortical growth over an extended period of time, referred to as the balloon model theory, in order to describe the variations in human cognition that when abnormally defected, can lead to psychiatric conditions like schizophrenia. The balloon model theory describes cortical growth as a mechanism similar to an expanding balloon, where stretching of the myelin to the surface disentangles neighboring neuronal columns and enables the affected cortex to better differentiate signals. Cortical growth is affected by genetics, environment, nutrition, and time. Human life history is unique because it delays the end of brain growth until the third decade of life, which allows environmental factors to exert influence, via balloon-like cortical growth and stretching, to impose much greater variability and plasticity in the final outcome of brain maturation. However, the increase of variability in brain maturation outcomes also has increased humans' susceptibility for disorders like schizophrenia. The onset of schizophrenia usually occurs between the ages of 16-30, and regions of the brain that mature last, including the frontal and temporal lobes, show more variable in maturation outcome and are also highly associated with symptoms of schizophrenia, as opposed to brain regions that develop earlier, such as the motor and somatosensory cortices. Thus, humans' collaborative evolution of functional asymmetry in the neocortex, improvement of fatty acid metabolism, and unique cortical growth maturation has been a driving force for the development of our variable complex cognition, but has left us susceptible for developing extreme variants in the form of mental disorders.

Sexual Selection Hypothesis

This hypothesis builds upon Crespi and Badcock's imprinted brain theory of autism and psychosis by suggesting that the behavioral traits associated with autism and schizophrenia have been beneficial for individual reproductive, mating, and parental strategies; and therefore, have been maintained throughout the human population via sexual selection. Under this hypothesis, autistic- and schizotypy-like traits exist as diametric opposites joined on the same spectrum of normal cognition, and most people display moderate degrees of one or both types of traits. When the spectrum of traits intertwine with the dynamics of genomic imprinting and principles of sexual selection within the context of bipaternal investment patterns, traits act as ornaments of mating behavior. Whereas autistic-like traits are selected for based on their display of mechanistic and practical intelligence for obtaining resources that indicate support for a long-term relationship, schizotypy-traits demonstrate verbal and artistic creativity that indicate strong genetic fitness for a short-term mating strategy. Therefore, variation in different cognitive traits remain adaptive life-history, reproductive, and paternal strategies according local ecological conditions and personal characteristics. Although the hypothesis proposes that the cognitive traits do not originate by means of sexual selection and likely evolved for reasons unrelated to mating, the behavioral effects dictated by the genetic autistic- and schizotypy-traits remain varied in the environment and remain under selection; only extreme variants of either of the traits result in their respective clinical condition.

Evolutionary Advantage

Creativity is an essential tool for human development and survival. Schizophrenia is more than a tragic risk for creative people: Its persistence in the gene pool is essential. It is there "because of shared genetic linkages to creativity. "Schizotypal thinking is often viewed as sharing features with creative thought, such as cognitive flexibility and divergent thinking via unusual but meaningful associations. These commonalities, coupled with the observed heritability of both constructs, suggest that there may be genetic factors common to both creativity and schizophrenia." . There are many creative and famous people with schizophrenia.

Paranoid Schizophrenia

Paranoid schizophrenia, also called schizophrenia, paranoid type, is a sub-type of schizophrenia as defined in the Diagnostic and Statistical Manual of Mental Disorders, DSM-IV code 295.30. It has been the most common type of schizophrenia. Schizophrenia is defined as "a chronic mental disorder in which a person loses touch with reality (psychosis)." Schizophrenia is divided into subtypes based on the "predominant symptomatology at the time of evaluation." The clinical picture is dominated by relatively stable and often persecutory delusions that are usually accompanied by hallucinations, particularly of the auditory variety (hearing voices), and perceptual disturbances. These symptoms can have a huge effect on functioning and can negatively affect quality of life. Paranoid schizophrenia is a lifelong disease, but with proper treatment, a person with the illness can attain a higher quality of life.

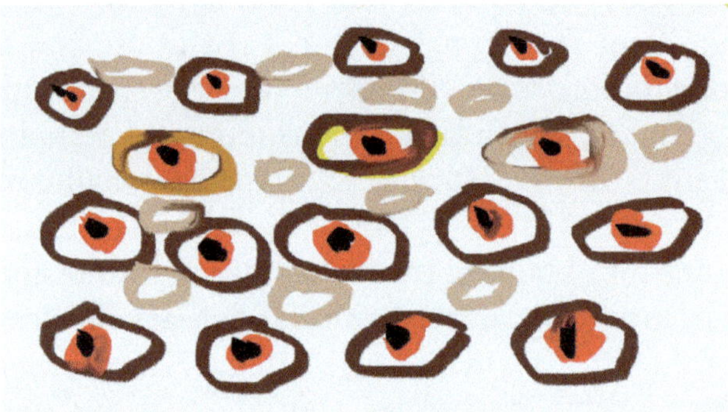

A work of outsider art made by a person with paranoid schizophrenia

Although paranoid schizophrenia is defined by those two symptoms, it is also defined by a lack of certain symptoms (negative symptoms). The following symptoms are not prominent: "disorganized speech, disorganized or catatonic behavior, or flat or inappropriate affect." Those symptoms are present in another form of schizophrenia, disorganized-type schizophrenia. The criteria for diagnosing paranoid schizophrenia must be present from at least one to six months. This helps to differentiate schizophrenia from other diseases, such as bipolar disorder.

Paranoid schizophrenia is defined in the Diagnostic and Statistical Manual of Mental Disorders, 4th Edition, but it was dropped from the 5th Edition. The American Psychiatric Association (APA) chose to eliminate schizophrenia subtypes because they had "limited diagnostic stability, low reliability, and poor validity." The symptoms and lack of symptoms that were being used to categorize the different subtypes of schizophrenia were not concrete enough to be able to be diagnosed. The APA also believed that the subtypes of schizophrenia should be removed because "they did not appear to help with providing better targeted treatment, or predicting treatment response." Targeted treatment and treatment response vary from patient to patient, depending on his or her symptoms. It is more beneficial, therefore, to look at the severity of the symptoms when considering treatment options.

Symptoms

Paranoid schizophrenia manifests itself in an array of symptoms. Common symptoms for paranoid schizophrenia include auditory hallucinations (hearing voices) and paranoid delusions (believing everyone is out to cause the sufferer harm). However, two of the symptoms separate this form of schizophrenia from other forms.

One criterion for separating paranoid schizophrenia from other types is delusion. A delusion is a belief that is held strong even when the evidence shows otherwise. Some common delusions associated with paranoid schizophrenia include, "believing that the government is monitoring every move you make, or that a co-worker is poisoning your lunch." In all but rare cases, these beliefs are irrational, and can cause the person holding them to behave abnormally. Another frequent type of delusion is a delusion of grandeur, or the "fixed, false belief that one possesses superior qualities such as genius, fame, omnipotence, or wealth." Common ones include, "the belief that you can fly, that you're famous, or that you have a relationship with a famous person."

Another criterion present in patients with paranoid schizophrenia is auditory hallucinations, in which the person hears voices or sounds that are not really present. The patient will sometimes hear multiple voices and the voices can either be talking to the patient or to one another. These voices that the patient hears can influence them to behave in a particular manner. Researchers at the Mayo Foundation for Medical Education and Research provide the following description: "They [the voices] may make ongoing criticisms of what you're thinking or doing, or make cruel comments about your real or imagined faults. Voices may also command you to do things that can be harmful to yourself or to others." A patient exhibiting these auditory hallucinations may be observed talking to themself because the person believes that the voices are actually present.

Early diagnosis is critical for the successful treatment of schizophrenia.

Diagnosis

The DSM-IV criteria (note there may be new criteria for the condition under the DSM-5) for the diagnosis of schizophrenia require the presence of symptoms for certain periods of time in order to successfully diagnose a person with schizophrenia. A person must exhibit two or more core symptoms for a minimum of one month, such as delusions, hallucinations, disorganized speech, grossly disorganized or catatonic behavior, or negative symptoms. There also must be significant impairment for the person at work, with academic performance, interpersonal relationships, and the ability to take care of oneself. These symptoms must continue for a minimum of six months with the first symptoms continuing for at least one month. Paranoid schizophrenia is differentiated by the presence of hallucinations and delusions involving the perception of persecution or grandiosity in one's beliefs about the world.

People with paranoid schizophrenia are often more articulate or "normal" seeming than other people with schizophrenia, such as hebephrenia-afflicted individuals. The diagnosis of paranoid schizophrenia is given with the presence of bizarre delusions or hallucinations that defy the natural laws of basic logical thought processes, or thought disorders and withdrawal due to these thoughts and delusions. The paranoid subset of schizophrenia tends to have a better prognosis than other subtypes (hebephrenic and simple in particular) as the intellect and personality are relatively preserved, thus enabling a greater degree of cognitive and interpersonal functioning.

With the removal of the subtypes of schizophrenia in DSM-5, paranoid schizophrenia will no longer be used as a diagnostic category. If a person is exhibiting symptoms of schizophrenia, including symptoms of paranoid type, they will simply be diagnosed with schizophrenia and will be treated with antipsychotics based on their individual symptoms.

Prevention

According to the Mayo Clinic, it is best to start receiving treatment for paranoid schizophrenia as early as possible and to maintain the treatment throughout life. Continuing treatment will help keep the serious symptoms under control and allow the person to lead a more fulfilling life. One cannot reduce the risk of developing paranoid schizophrenia. This illness is typically unpreventable.

It has a strong hereditary component with a first degree parent or sibling. There is some possibility that there are environmental influences including "prenatal exposure to a viral infection, low oxygen levels during birth (from prolonged labor or premature birth), exposure to a virus during infancy, early parental loss or separation, and verbal, physical or sexual abuse in childhood". Eliminating any of these factors could help reduce an individual's future risk of developing paranoid schizophrenia.

Treatment

Paranoid schizophrenia is an illness that typically requires lifelong treatment with neuroleptics to allow someone to have a relatively stable and normal lifestyle. In order to be successfully treated, a person with schizophrenia should seek help from family or primary care doctors, psychiatrists, psychotherapists, pharmacists, family members, case workers, psychiatric nurses, or social workers, provided he or she is not unable to do so, due to many people with schizophrenia having the inability to accept their condition. Non-compliance with neuroleptics may also occur if the patient considers the side effects (such as extrapyramidal symptoms) to be more debilitating than the condition itself. The main options that are offered for the treatment of paranoid schizophrenia are the following: neuroleptics, psychotherapy, hospitalization, electroconvulsive therapy, and vocational skills training.

There are many different types of disorders that have similar symptoms to paranoid schizophrenia. There are tests that psychiatrists perform to achieve a correct diagnosis. They include "psychiatric evaluation, in which the doctor or psychiatrist will ask a series of questions about the patient's symptoms, psychiatric history, and family history of mental health problems; medical history and exam, in which the doctor will ask about one's personal and family health history and will also perform a complete physical examination to check for medical issues that could be causing or contributing to the problem; laboratory tests in which the doctor will order simple blood and urine tests can rule out other medical causes of symptoms". There are side effects associated with antipsychotic medication. Neuroleptics can cause high blood pressure and high cholesterol. Many people who take them exhibit weight gain and have a higher risk of developing diabetes.

History

Since the early 19th century, schizophrenia has been recognized as a psychiatric disorder. It was described in 1883 by Emil Kraepelin as dementia praecox, or the premature deterioration of the brain. It was believed to be untreatable and unstoppable. At that time, very few people were diagnosed with dementia praecox due to the small range of symptoms recognized specifically as signs of this disorder. Years later, Eugen Bleuler coined the term *schizophrenia*, which literally means "split mind".

Bleuler thought that the disorder caused a person to no longer be able to function mentally due to a lack of mental associations between thought, language, emotions, memory and problem solving, due to the splitting of their mind. Eventually, the broad diagnosis of schizophrenia was narrowed to a set of specific types of symptoms that were necessary in order to diagnose the disorder, and was also split into several different types: paranoid, disorganized, and catatonic (each with its own specific symptoms), along with undifferentiated and residual schizophrenia, which are a combination or very few residual symptoms of schizophrenia.

During World War II, the Nazi Party attempted to eradicate schizophrenia by compulsory sterilization and the killing of psychiatric patients.

As of 2013, with the publication of the new DSM-5, the different subtypes of schizophrenia are no longer specified or differentiated from schizophrenia in the manual. Instead, schizophrenia is viewed as one mental disorder with an array of different symptoms. Treatment for people suffering from schizophrenia is based on the type of symptoms that are exhibited in each individual case.

Disorganized Schizophrenia

Disorganized schizophrenia, also known as hebephrenia, is a subtype of schizophrenia, although it is not recognized in the latest version of the *Diagnostic and Statistical Manual of Mental Disorders*.

Disorganized schizophrenia is thought to be an extreme expression of the *disorganization syndrome* that has been hypothesized to be one aspect of a three-factor model of symptoms in schizophrenia, the other factors being *reality distortion* (involving delusions and hallucinations) and *psychomotor poverty* (lack of speech, lack of spontaneous movement and various aspects of blunting of emotion).

Presentation

The condition is also known as hebephrenia, named after the Greek term for "a boy" - *hebeos,* and possibly the ancient Greek goddess of youth, Hebe, daughter of Hera. The term refers to the ostensibly more prominent appearance of the disorder in persons around puberty.

The prominent characteristics of this form are disorganized behavior and speech, including loosened associations and schizophasia ("word salad"), and flat or inappropriate affect. In addition, psychiatrists must rule out any possible sign of catatonic schizophrenia.

The most prominent features of disorganized schizophrenia are not delusions and hallucinations, as they are in paranoid schizophrenia, although fragmentary delusions, unsystemized and often hypochondriacal, and hallucinations may be present. A person with disorganized schizophrenia may also experience behavioral disorganization, which may impair his or her ability to carry out daily activities such as showering or eating.

The emotional responses of such people often seem strange or inappropriate. Inappropriate facial responses may be common, and behavior is sometimes described as 'silly', such as inappropriate laughter. Sometimes, there is a complete lack of emotion, including anhedonia (the lack of pleasure), and avolition (a lack of motivation). Some of these features are also present in other types of schizophrenia, but they are most prominent in disorganized schizophrenia.

Treatment

This form of schizophrenia is typically associated with early onset (often between the ages of 15 and 25 years) and is thought to have a poor prognosis because of the rapid development of negative symptoms and decline in social functioning.

Use of electroconvulsive therapy has been proposed; however, the effectiveness after treatment is in question.

Pediatric Schizophrenia

Pediatric schizophrenia (also known as childhood schizophrenia, childhood-onset schizophrenia, and early-onset schizophrenia) is a type of mental disorder that is characterized by degeneration of thinking, motor, and emotional processes, with onset before age 18 (early onset) or before age 13 (very early onset). The disease presents symptoms such as auditory and visual hallucinations, strange thoughts or feelings, and abnormal behavior, profoundly impacting the child's ability to function and sustain normal interpersonal relationships. It typically presents after the age of seven. About 50% of young children diagnosed with schizophrenia experience severe neuropsychiatric symptoms. Diagnostic criteria are similar to those of adult schizophrenia. Diagnosis is based on behavior observed by caretakers and, in some cases depending on age, self reports.

Schizophrenia has no definite cause; however, certain risk factors such as family history seem to correlate. There is no known cure, but childhood schizophrenia is controllable with the help of behavioral therapies and medications.

Signs and Symptoms

Schizophrenia is a psychiatric disorder that is expressed in abnormal mental functions and disturbed behavior.

The signs and symptoms of childhood schizophrenia are nearly the same as adult-onset schizophrenia. Some of the earliest signs that a young child may develop schizophrenia are lags in language and motor development. Some children engage in activities such as flapping the arms or rocking, and may appear anxious, confused, or disruptive on a regular basis. Children may experience symptoms such as hallucinations, but these are often difficult to differentiate from just normal imagination or child play. It is often difficult for children to describe their hallucinations or delusions, making early-onset schizophrenia especially difficult to diagnose in the earliest stages. The cognitive abilities of children with schizophrenia may also often be lacking, with 20% of patients showing borderline or full intellectual disability.

Very early-onset schizophrenia refers to onset before the age of thirteen. The prodromal phase, which precedes psychotic symptoms, is characterized by deterioration in school performance, social withdrawal, disorganized or unusual behavior, a decreased ability to perform daily activities, a deterioration in self-care skills, bizarre hygiene and eating behaviors, changes in affect, a lack of impulse control, hostility and aggression, and lethargy.

Auditory hallucinations are the most common positive symptom in children. A child's auditory hallucinations may include voices that are conversing with each other or voices that are speaking directly to the children themselves. Many children with auditory hallucinations believe that if they do not listen to the voices, the voices will harm them or someone else. Tactile and visual hallucinations seem relatively rare. Delusions are reported in more than half of children with schizophrenia, but they are usually less complex than those of adults.

Diagnosis

The same criteria are used to diagnose children and adults, but diagnosis of children is more challenging. Diagnosis is based on reports by parents or caretakers, teachers, school officials, and others close to the child.

A professional who believes a child has schizophrenia usually conducts a series of tests to rule out other causes of behavior, and pinpoint a diagnosis. Three different types of exams are performed: physical, laboratory, and psychological. Physical exams usually cover the basic assessments, including but not limited to; height, weight, blood pressure, and checking all vital signs to make sure the child is healthy. Laboratory tests include electroencephalogram EEG screening and brain imaging scans. Blood tests are used to rule out alcohol or drug effects, and thyroid hormone levels are tested to rule out hyper- or hypothyroidism. A psychologist or psychiatrist talks to a child about their thoughts, feelings, and behavior patterns. They also inquire about the severity of the symptoms, and the effects they have on the child's daily life. They may also discuss thoughts of suicide or self-harm in these one-on-one sessions. Some symptoms that may be looked at are early language delays, early motor development delays and school problems.

Cause

There is no known single cause or causes of schizophrenia, however, it is a heritable disorder.

Genetic

There is "considerable overlap" in the genetics of childhood-onset and adult-onset schizophrenia, but in childhood-onset schizophrenia there is a higher number of "rare allelic variants". An important gene for adolescent-onset schizophrenia is the catechol-O-methyltransferase gene, a gene that regulates dopamine. Children with schizophrenia have an increase in genetic deletions or duplication mutations and some have a specific mutation called 22q11 deletion syndrome, which accounts for up to 2% of cases.

Neuroanatomical

Neuroimaging studies have found differences between medicated schizophrenic brains and neurotypical brains, though research does not know the cause of the difference. In childhood-onset schizophrenia, there appears to be a faster reduction of gray matter.

Epidemiology

Schizophrenia disorders in children are rare. Boys are twice as likely to be diagnosed with childhood schizophrenia. People have been and still are reluctant to diagnose schizophrenia early on, primarily due to the stigma attached to it.

Prevention

Research efforts are focusing on prevention in identifying early signs from relatives with associated disorders similar with schizophrenia and those with prenatal and birth complications. Prevention has been an ongoing challenge because early signs of the disorder are similar to those of other disorders. Also, some of the schizophrenic related symptoms are often found in children without schizophrenia or any other diagnosable disorder.

Treatment

Current methods in treating early-onset schizophrenia follow a similar approach to the treatment of adult schizophrenia. Although modes of treatment in this population is largely understudied, the use of antipsychotic medication is commonly the first line of treatment in addressing symptoms. Recent literature has failed to determine if typical or atypical antipsychotics are most effective in reducing symptoms and improving outcomes. When weighing treatment options, it is necessary to consider the averse effects of various medications used to treat schizophrenia and the potential implications of these effects on development.

Prognosis

An early or very-early diagnosis of schizophrenia leads to a worse prognosis than other psychotic disorders. The primary area that children with schizophrenia must adapt to is their social surroundings. It has been found, however, that early-onset schizophrenia carried a more severe prognosis than later-onset schizophrenia. Regardless of treatment, children diagnosed with schizophrenia at an early age suffer diminished social skills, such as educational and vocational abilities.

The grey matter in the cerebral cortex of the brain shrinks over time in people with schizophrenia; the question of whether antipsychotic medication exacerbates or causes this has been controversial. A 2015 meta-analysis found that there is a positive correlation between the cumulative amount of first generation antipsychotics taken by people with schizophrenia and the amount of grey matter loss, and a negative correlation with the cumulative amount of second-generation antipsychotics taken.

History

Until the late nineteenth century, children were often diagnosed as suffering from psychosis like schizophrenia, but instead were said to suffer from "pubescent" or "developmental" insanity. Through the 1950s, childhood psychosis began to become more and more common, and psychiatrists began to take a deeper look into the issue.

By the 1960s, "childhood schizophrenia" became known as a "heterogeneous mixture" of different disorders, such as autism, symbiotic psychosis, and dementia infantilis. Childhood schizophrenia was not directly added to the DSM until 1968, when it was added to the DSM-II, which set forth diagnostic criteria similar to that of adult schizophrenia. "Schizophrenia, childhood type" was a DSM-II diagnosis with diagnostic code 295.8*. It's equivalent to "schizophrenic reaction, childhood type" (000-x28) in DSM-I (1952).

The diagnosis of schizophrenia was often given to children who by today's standards would be diagnosed as having of autism or pervasive developmental disorder. This may be because the onset of schizophrenia is gradual, with symptoms relating developmental difficulties or abnormalities appearing before psychotic symptoms.

Mechanisms of Schizophrenia

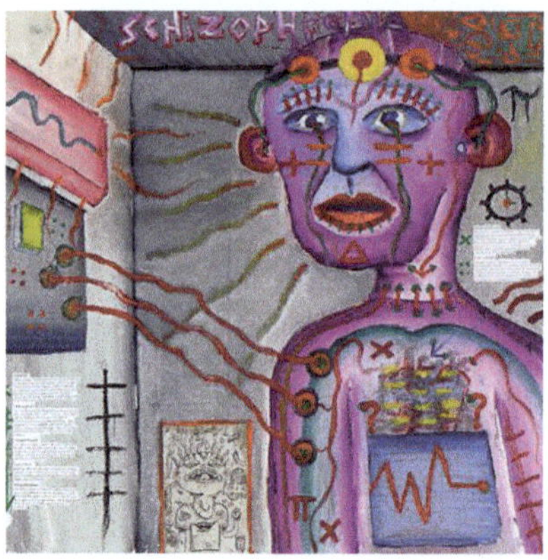

Artistic view of what the world feels like with schizophrenia

The underlying mechanisms of schizophrenia, a mental disorder characterized by a disintegration of the processes of thinking and of emotional responsiveness, are complex. A number of theories attempt to explain the link between altered brain function and schizophrenia, the most important of which are the dopamine hypothesis and the glutamate hypothesis. Note that these theories are separate from the causes of schizophrenia, which deal with actual starting points of the illness instead, e.g. genetic and environmental factors. The current theories attempt to explain how changes in brain functioning can contribute to symptoms of the disease.

Pathophysiology

The exact pathophysiology of schizophrenia remains poorly understood. Since the coining of schizophrenia by Eugene Bleuler in 1908, a variety of theories have been proposed concerning its underlying pathophysiology. The most commonly supported theories are the dopamine hypothesis and the glutamate hypothesis. More recent theories center around specific dysfunction of interneurons, abnormalities in the immune system, abnormalities in myelination, and oxidative stress.

Dopamine Dysfunction

An influential theory, known as the "dopamine hypothesis of schizophrenia", proposes that a malfunction involving dopamine pathways is therefore the cause of (the positive symptoms of) schizophrenia, with a particular focus on the function of dopamine in the mesolimbic pathway of the brain. This focus largely resulted from the accidental finding that a drug group which blocks dopamine function, known as the phenothiazines, could reduce psychotic symptoms. It is also supported by the fact that amphetamines, which trigger the release of dopamine, may exacerbate the psychotic symptoms in schizophrenia.

The theory proposes that excess activation of D_2 receptors underlies (the positive symptoms of) schizophrenia. Although postulated for about 20 years based on the D_2 blockade effect common to all antipsychotics, it was not until the mid-1990s that PET and SPET imaging studies provided supporting evidence. This explanation is now thought to be simplistic, partly because newer antipsychotic medication (called atypical antipsychotic medication) can be equally effective as older medication (called typical antipsychotic medication), but also affects serotonin function and may have slightly less of a dopamine blocking effect.

Evidence for this theory includes findings that the potency of many antipsychotics is correlated with their affinity to dopamine D_2 receptors; and the exacerbatory effects of a dopamine agonist (amphetamine) and a dopamine beta hydroxylase inhibitor (disulfiram) on schizophrenia; and post-mortem studies initially suggested increased density of dopamine D_2 receptors in the striatum. Such high levels of D_2 receptors intensify brain signals and can exacerbate positive symptoms (*i.e.* hallucinations and paranoia) in schizophrenia. Impaired glutamate (a neurotransmitter which directs neuron to pass along an impulse) activity appears to be another source of schizophrenia symptoms.

The importance of the dopamine theory has been further strengthened by the finding for common variant in the dopamine D2 receptor as candidate loci for the disease, as identified by the large genome-wide association study which included over 35,000 cases and over 110,000 controls.

Exactly how dopamine dysregulation can contribute to schizophrenia symptoms remains unclear. Some studies have suggested that disruption of the auditory thalamocortical projections give rise to hallucinations, while dysregulated corticostriatal circuitry and reward circuitry in the form of aberrant salience can give rise to delusions.

Glutamate Abnormalities

Beside the dopamine hypothesis, interest has also focused on the neurotransmitter glutamate and the reduced function of the NMDA glutamate receptor in the pathophysiology of schizophrenia. This has largely been suggested by lower levels of glutamate receptors found in postmortem brains of people previously diagnosed with schizophrenia and the discovery that the glutamate blocking drugs such as phencyclidine and ketamine can mimic the symptoms and cognitive problems associated with the condition.

The fact that reduced glutamate function is linked to poor performance on tests requiring frontal lobe and hippocampal function and that glutamate can affect dopamine function, all of which have been implicated in schizophrenia, have suggested an important mediating (and possibly causal) role of glutamate pathways in schizophrenia. Positive symptoms fail however to respond to glutamatergic medication.

Reduced mRNA and protein expression of several NMDA receptor subunits has also been reported in postmortem brains from patients with schizophrenia.

The large genome-wide association study mentioned above has supported glutamate abnormalities for schizophrenia, reporting several mutations in genes related to glutamatergic neurotransmission, such as GRIN2A, GRIA1, SRR, and GRM3.

Interneuron Dysfunction

A novel hypothesis concerning the pathophysiology of schizophrenia, one that closely relates to the glutamate hypothesis, is one that evolves around dysfunction of interneurons in the brain. Interneurons in the brain are GABAergic and local, and function mainly through the inhibition of other cells. One type of interneuron, the fast-spiking, parvalbumin-positive interneuron, has been suggested to play a key role in schizophrenia pathophysiology.

Early studies have identified decreases in GAD67 mRNA and protein in post-mortem brains from schizophrenia patients compared to controls. Interestingly, these reductions were found in only a subset of cortical interneurons. Furthermore, GAD67 mRNA was completely undetectable in a subset of interneurons also expressing parvalbumin. Levels of parvalbumin protein and mRNA were also found to be lower in patient brains in various regions in the brain. Actual numbers of parvalbumin interneurons have been found to be unchanged in these studies, however, except for a single study showing a decrease in parvalbumin interneurons in the hippocampus. Finally, excitatory synapse density is lower selectively on parvalbumin interneurons in schizophrenia and predicts the activity-dependent down-regulation of parvalbumin and GAD67. Together, this suggests that parvalbumin interneurons are somehow specifically affected in the disease.

Several studies have tried to assess levels in GABA *in vivo* in the patients with schizophrenia, but these findings have remained inconclusive.

EEG studies have indirectly also pointed to interneuron dysfunction in schizophrenia. These studies have pointed to abnormalities in oscillatory activity in schizophrenia, particularly in the gamma band (30–80 Hz). Interestingly, gamma band activity appears to originate from intact functioning parvalbumin-positive interneuron. Together with the post-mortem findings, these EEG abnormalities point to a role for dysfunctional parvalbumin interneurons in schizophrenia.

The largest meta-analysis on copy-number variations (CNVs), structural abnormalities in the form of genetic deletions or duplications, to date for schizophenia, published in 2015, was the first genetic evidence for the broad involvement of GABAergic neurotransmission.

Myelination Abnormalities

Another hypothesis states that abnormalities in myelination are a core pathophysiology of schizophrenia. This theory originated from structural imaging studies, who found that white matter regions, in addition to grey matter regions, showed volumetric reductions in patients with schizophrenia. In addition, gene expression studies have shown abnormalities in myelination and oligodendrocytes in post-mortem brains of schizophrenia patients. Furthermore, oligodendrocyte numbers appear to be reduced in several post-mortem studies.

It has been suggested that myelination abnormalities could originate from impaired maturation of oligodendrocyte precursor cells, as these have been found to be intact in schizophrenia brains.

Immune System Abnormalities

Another hypothesis postulates that inflammation and immune system abnormalities could play a central role in the disease. Abnormal immune system development may help explain roles of environmental effect such as prenatal hazards, post-pubertal onset, stress, climate, and infections, in addition to genetic effects. The immune hypotheses is supported by findings of high levels of immune markers in the blood of schizophrenia patients. High levels of immune markers have also been associated with having more severe psychotic symptoms. Furthermore, a meta-analysis of genome-wide association studies discovered that 129 out of 136 single-nucleotide polymorphisms (SNP) significantly associated with schizophrenia were located in the major histocompatibility complex region of the genome.

A recent systematic review investigating neuroinflammatory markers in post-mortem schizophrenia brains has shown quite some variability, with some studies showing alterations in various markers but others failing to find any differences.

Oxidative Stress

A theory that has gained more support in recent years is that a large role is played in the disease by oxidative stress. Redox dysregulation in early development can potentially influence development of different cell types that have been shown to be impaired in the disease.

Oxidative stress has also been indicated through genetic studies into schizophrenia.

Oxidative stress has been shown to affect maturation of oligodendrocytes, the myelinating cell types in the brain, potentially underlying the white matter abnormalities found in the brain.

Furthermore, oxidative stress could also influence the development of GABAergic interneurons, which have also been found to be dysregulated in schizophrenia.

Structural Abnormalities

Beside theories concerning the functional mechanism underlying the disease, structural findings have been identified as well using a wide range of imaging techniques. Studies have tended to show various subtle average differences in the volume of certain areas of brain structure between people with and without diagnoses of schizophrenia, although it has become increasingly clear that no single pathological neuropsychological or structural neuroanatomic profile exists.

MRI

Structural imaging studies have extensively reported differences in the size and structure of certain brain areas in schizophrenia.

The largest combined neuroimaging study with over 2000 patients and 2500 controls has replicated these previous findings. Here, the authors found volumetric increases in the lateral ventricles (+18%), caudate and pallidum, and extensive decreases in the hippocampus (-4%), thalamus, amygdala and nucleus accumbens. Together, this indicates that extensive changes occur in brains in patients suffering from schizophrenia.

A 2006 meta-analysis of MRI studies found that whole brain and hippocampal volume are reduced and that ventricular volume is increased in patients with a first psychotic episode relative to healthy controls. The average volumetric changes in these studies are however close to the limit of detection by MRI methods, so it remains to be determined whether schizophrenia is a neurodegenerative process that begins at about the time of symptom onset, or whether it is better characterised as a neurodevelopmental process that produces abnormal brain volumes at an early age. In first episode psychosis typical antipsychotics like haloperidol were associated with significant reductions in gray matter volume, whereas atypical antipsychotics like olanzapine were not. Studies in non-human primates found gray and white matter reductions for both typical and atypical antipsychotics.

Abnormal findings in the prefrontal cortex, temporal cortex and anterior cingulate cortex are found before the first onset of schizophrenia symptoms. These regions are the regions of structural deficits found in schizophrenia and first-episode patients. Positive symptoms, such as thoughts of being persecuted, were found to be related to the medial prefrontal cortex, amygdala, and hippocampus region. Negative symptoms were found to be related to the ventrolateral prefrontal cortex and ventral striatum.

Ventricular and third ventricle enlargement, abnormal functioning of the amygdala, hippocampus, parahippocampal gyrus, neocortical temporal lobe regions, frontal lobe, prefontal gray matter, orbitofrontal areas, parietal lobs abnormalities and subcortical abnormalities including the cavum septi pellucidi, basal ganglia, corpus callosum, thalamus and cerebellar abnormalities. Such abnormalities usually present in the form of loss of volume.

Most schizophrenia studies have found average reduced volume of the left medial temporal lobe and left superior temporal gyrus, and half of studies have revealed deficits in certain areas of the frontal gyrus, parahippocampal gyrus and temporal gyrus. However, at variance with some findings in individuals with chronic schizophrenia significant group differences of temporal lobe and amygdala volumes are not shown in first-episode patients on average.

Finally, MRI studies utilizing modern cortical surface reconstruction techniques have shown widespread reduction in cerebral cortical thickness (i.e., "cortical thinning") in frontal and temporal regions and somewhat less widespread cortical thinning in occipital and parietal regions in patients with schizophrenia, relative to healthy control subjects. Moreover, one study decomposed cortical volume into its constituent parts, cortical surface area and cortical thickness, and reported widespread cortical volume reduction in schizophrenia, mainly driven by cortical thinning, but also reduced cortical surface area in smaller frontal, temporal, parietal and occipital cortical regions.

DTI

Diffusion tensor imaging (DTI) allows for the investigation of white matter more closely than traditional MRI. Over 300 DTI imaging studies have been published examining white matter abnormalities in schizophrenia. Although quite some variation has been found pertaining to the specific regions affected, the general consensus states a reduced fractional anisotropy in brains from patients with schizophrenia versus controls. Importantly, these differences between patients and controls could potentially be attributed to lifestyle effects, medication effects etc. Therefore, more recently several studies have been perform in first-onset schizophrenia patients that have never recent any medication, so-called medication-naive subjects. These studies, although still few in number, also found reduced fractional anisotropy in patient brains compared to control brains. As with earlier findings, abnormalities can be found throughout the brain, although the corpus callous seemed to be most commonly effected.

CT

Computed Tomography scans of schizophrenic brains show several pathologies. The brain ventricles are enlarged as compared to normal brains. The ventricles hold cerebrospinal fluid (CSF) and enlarged ventricles indicate a loss of brain volume. Additionally, schizophrenic brains have widened sulci as compared to normal brains, also with increased CSF volumes and reduced brain volume.

Functional Abnormalities

PET

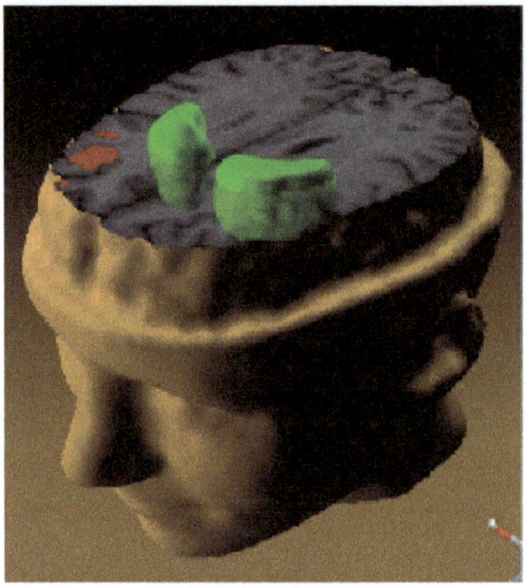

Data from a PET study suggests that the less the frontal lobes are activated (red) during a working memory task, the greater the increase in abnormal dopamine activity in the striatum (green), thought to be related to the neurocognitive deficits in schizophrenia.

PET scan findings in patients with schizophrenia indicate cerebral blood flow decreases in the left parahippocampal region. PET scans also show a reduced ability to metabolize glucose in the thalamus and frontal cortex. PET scans also show involvement of the medial part of the left temporal lobe and the limbic and frontal systems as suffering from developmental abnormality. PET scans show thought disorders stem from increased flow in the frontal and temporal regions while delusions and hallucinations were associated with reduced flow in the cingulate, left frontal, and temporal areas. PET scans done on patient who were actively having auditory hallucinations revealed increased blood flow in both thalami, left hippocampus, right striatum, parahippocampus, orbitofrontal, and cingulate areas.

In addition, a decrease in NAA uptake has been reported in the hippocampus and both the grey and white matter of the prefrontal cortex of those with schizophrenia. NAA may be an indicator of neural activity of number of viable neurons. however given methodological limitations and variance it is impossible to use this as a diagnostic method. Decreased PFC connectivity has also been observed. DOPA PET studies have confirmed an altered synthesis capacity of dopamine in the nigrostriatal system demonstrating a dopaminergic dysregulation.

Glutamate Hypothesis of Schizophrenia

The glutamate hypothesis of schizophrenia models the subset of pathologic mechanisms linked to glutamatergic signaling. The hypothesis was initially based on a set of clinical, neuropathological, and, later, genetic findings pointing at a hypofunction of glutamatergic signaling via NMDA receptors. While thought to be more proximal to the root causes of schizophrenia, it does not negate the dopamine hypothesis, and the two may be ultimately brought together by circuit-based models. The development of the hypothesis allowed for the integration of the GABAergic and oscillatory abnormalities into the converging disease model and made it possible to discover the causes of some disruptions.

Like the dopamine hypothesis, the development of the glutamate hypothesis developed from the observed effects of mind-altering drugs. However, where dopamine agonists can mimic positive symptoms with significant risks to brain structures during and after use, NMDA antagonists mimic some positive and negative symptoms with less brain harm. Likely, both dopaminergic and glutaminergic abnormalities are implicated in schizophrenia, from a profound alteration in the function of the chemical synapses, as well as electrical synaptic irregularities. These form a portion of the complex constellation of factors, neurochemically, psychologically, psychosocially, and structurally, which result in schizophrenia.

The Role of Heteromer Formation

Alteration in the expression, distribution, autoregulation, and prevalence of specific glutamate heterodimers alters relative levels of paired G proteins to the heterodimer-forming glutamate receptor in question.

Namely: 5HT2A and mGlu2 form a dimer which mediates psychotomimetic and ethenogenin effects of psychedelics; as such this receptor is of interest in schizophrenia. Agonists at either constituent receptor may modulate the other receptor allosterically; e.g. glutamate-dependent signaling via mGlu2 may modulate 5HT2A-ergic activity. Equillibrium between mGlu2/5HT2A is altered against tendency towards of psychosis by nueroleptic-pattern 5HT2A antagonists and mGlu2 agonists; both display antipsychotic activity. AMPA, the most widely distributed receptor in the brain, is a tetrameric ionotropic receptor; alterations in equillibrium between constituent subunits are seen in mGlu2/5HT2A antagonist (antipsychotic) administration- GluR2 is seen to be upregulated in the PFC while GluR1 downregulates in response to antipsychotic administration.

Reelin abnormalities may also be involved in the pathogenesis of schizophrenia via a glutamate-dependent mechanism. Reelin expression deficits are seen in schizophrenia, and reelin enhances expression of AMPA and NMDA alike. As such deficits in these two ionotropic glutamate receptors may be partially explained by altered reelin cascades. Neuregulin 1 deficits may also be involved in glutaminergic hypofunction as NRG1 hypofunction leads to schizophrenia-pattern behavior in mice; likely due in part to reduced NMDA signaling via Src suppression.

The Role of Synaptic Pruning

Various neurotrophic factors dysregulate in schizophrenia and other mental illnesses, namely BDNF; expression of which is lowered in schizophrenia as well as in major depression and bipolar disorder. BDNF regulates in an AMPA-dependent mechanism - AMPA and BDNF alike are critical mediators of growth cone survival. NGF, another neurotrophin involved in maintinence of synaptic plasticity is similarly seen in deficit.

Dopaminergic excess, classically understood to result in schizophrenia, puts oxidative load on neurons; leading to inflammatory response and microglia activation. Similarly, toxoplasmosis infection in the CNS (positively correlated to schizophrenia) activates inflammatory cascades, also leading to microglion activation. The lipoxygenase-5 inhibitor minocycline has been seen to be marginally effective in halting schizophrenia progression. One of such inflammatory cascades' downstream transcriptional target, NF-kb, is observed to have altered expression in schizophrenia.

In addition, CB2 is one of the most widely distributed glial cell-expressed receptors, downregulation of this inhibitory receptor may increase global synaptic pruning activity. While difference in expression or distribution is observed, when the CB2 receptor is knocked out in mice, schizophreniform behaviors manifest. This may deregulate synaptic pruning processes in a tachyphlaxis mechanism wherein immediate excess CB2 activity leads to phosphorylation of the receptor via GIRK, resultant in b-arrestin-dependent internalization and subsequent trafficking to the proteasome for degradation.

The Role of Endogenous Antagonists

Alterations in production of endogenous NMDA antagonists such as agmatine and kyenurenic acid have been shown in schizophrenia. Deficit in NMDA activity produces psychotomimetic effects, though it remains to be seen if the blockade of NMDA via these agents is causative or actually mimetic of patterns resultant from monoaminergic disruption.

AMPA, the most widely distributed receptor in the brain, mediates long term potentiation via activity-dependent modulation of AMPA density. GluR1 subunit-containing AMPA receptors are Ca2+ permiable while GluR2/3 subunit-positive receptors are nearly impermeable to calcium ions. In the regulated pathway, GluR1 dimers populate the synapse at a rate proportional to NMDA-ergic Ca2+ influx. In the constitutative pathway, GluR2/3 dimers populate the synapse at a steady state.

This forms a positive feedback loop, where a small trigger impulse degating NMDA from Mg2+ pore blockade results in calcium influx, this calcium influx then triggers trafficking of GluR1-containing(Ca2+ permeable) subunits to the PSD, such trafficking of GluR1-positive AMPA to the postsynaptic neuron allows for upmodulation of the postsynaptic neuron's calcium influx in response to presynaptic calcium influx. Robust negative feedback at NMDA from kyenurenic acid, magnesium, zinc, and agmatine prevents runaway feedback.

Misregulation of this pathway would sympathetically dysregulate LTP via disruption of NMDA. Such alteration in LTP may play a role, specifically in negative symptoms of schizophrenia, in creation of more broad disruptions such as loss of brain volume; an effect of the disease which antidopaminergics actually worsen, rather than treat.

The Role of a7 Nicotinic

Anandamide, an endocannabinoid, is an a7 nicotinic antagonist. Cigarettes, consumed far out of proportion by schizophrenics, contain nornitrosonicotine; a potent a7 antagonist. This may indicate a7 pentameter excess as a causative factor, or possibly as a method of self-medication to combat antipsychotic side effects. Cannabidiol, a FAAH inhibitor, increases levels in anandamide and may have antipsychotic effect; though results are mixed here as anandamide also is a cannabinoid and as such displays some psychotomimetic effect. However, a7 nicotinic *agonists* have been indicated as potential treatments for schizophrenia, though evidence is somewhat contradictory there is indication a7 nAChR is somehow involved in the pathogenesis of schizophrenia.

The Role of 5-HT

This deficit in activation also results in a decrease in activity of 5-HT1A receptors in the raphe nucleus.(Bantick, Deakin, Grasby 2001) This serves to increase global serotonin levels, as 5-HT1A serves as an autoreceptor. The 5-HT1B receptor, also acting as an autoreceptor, specifically within the striatum, but also parts of basal ganglia then will inhibit serotonin release. This disinhibits frontal dopamine release. The local deficit of 5-HT within the striatum, basal ganglia, and prefrontal cortex causes a deficit of excitatory 5-HT6 signalling. This receptor is primarily GABAergic, as such, it causes an excess of glutamatergic, noradrenergic, dopaminergic, and cholinergic activity within the prefrontal cortex and the striatum. An excess of 5-HT7 signaling within the thalamus also creates too much excitatory transmission to the prefrontal cortex. Combined with another critical abnormality observed in schizoid patients: 5-HT2A dysfunction, this altered signalling cascade creates cortical, thus cognitive abnormalities. 5-HT2A allows a link between cortical, thus conscious, and the basal ganglia, unconscious. Axons from 5-HT2A neurons in layer V of the cerebral cortex reach the basal ganglia, forming a feedback loop. Signalling from layer V of the cerebral cortex to the basal ganglia alters 5-HT2C signalling. This feedback loop with 5-HT2A/5-HT2C is how the outer cortex layers can exert some control over our neuropeptides, specifically opioid peptides, oxytocin and vasopressin. This alteration in this limbic-layer V axis may create the profound change in social cognition (and sometimes cognition as a whole) that is observed in schizoid patients. However, genesis of the actual alterations is a much more complex phenomena.

The Role of Inhibitory Transmission

The cortico-basal galglia-thalamo-cortical loop is the source of the ordered input necessary for a higher level upper cortical loop. Feedback is controlled by the inhibitory potential of the cortices via the striatum. Through 5-HT2A efferents from layer V of the cortex transmission proceeds through the striatum into the globulus pallidus internal and substantia nigra pars compacta. This core input to the basal galglia is combined with input from the subthalamic nucleus. The only primarily dopaminergic pathway in this loop is a reciprocal connection from the substantia nigra pars reticulata to the striatum.

Dopaminergic drugs such as dopamine releasing agents and direct dopamine receptor agonists create alterations in this primarily GABAergic pathway via increased dopaminergic feedback from the substantia nigra pars compacta to the striatum. However, dopamine also modulates other cortical areas, namely the VTA; with efferents to the amygdala and locus coeruleus, likely modulating anxiety and paranoid aspects of psychotic experience. As such, the glutamate hypothesis is probably not an explanation of primary causative factors in positive psychosis, but rather might possibly be an explanation for negative symptoms.

Dopamine hypothesis of schizophrenia elaborattes upon the nature of abnormal lateral structures found in someone with a high risk for psychosis.

Altered Signalling Cascades

Again, thalamic input from layer V is a crucial factor in the functionality of the human brain. It allows the two sides to receive similar inputs, thus be able to perceive the same world. In psychosis, thalamic input loses much of its integrated character: hyperactive core feedback loops overwhelm the ordered output. This is due to excessive D2 and 5-HT2A activity. This alteration in input to the top and bottom of the cortex. The altered 5-HT signal cascade enhances the strength of excitatory thalamic input from layer V. This abnormality, enhancing the thalamic-cortical transmission cascade versus the corticostrriratal control, creates a feedback loop, resulting in abnormally strong basal ganglic output.

The root of psychosis(experiences that cannot be explained, even within their own mind) is when basal ganglic input to layer V overwhelms the inhibitory potential of the higher cortexies resulting from striatal transmission. When combined with the excess prefrontal, specifically orbitofrontal tranmsmission, from lthe hippocampus, this creates a brain prone to falling into self reinforcing belief.

However, given a specific environment, a person with this kind of brain(a human) can create a self-reinforcing pattern of maladaptive behavior, from the altered the layer II/III and III/I axises, from the disinhibited thalamic output. Rationality is impaired, primarily as response to the deficit of oxytocin and excess of vasopressin from the abnormal 5HT2C activity. An altered HPA axis, perhaps from xenohormones, drug use, or a genetic predisposition to altered adregenic and norepineprine signalling. Altered HPA axis, towards more cortisol activation is a primary pathological marker in seen many disorders.

Frontal cortex activity will be impaired, when combined with excess DA activity: the basis for the advancement of schizophrenia, but it is also the neurologic mechanism behind many other psychotic diseases as well.. Heredation of schizophrenia may even be a result of conspecific "refrigerator parenting" techniqes passed on though generations. However, the genetic component is the primary source of the neurological abnormalities which leave one prone to psychological disorders. Specifically, there is much overlap between bipolar disorder and schizophrenia, and other psychotic disorders.

Psychotic disorder is linked to excessive drug use, specifically dissociatives, psychedelics, stimulants, and marijuana.

Current State of Schizophrenia Treatment

Schizophrenia is now treated by medications known as antipsychotics (or neuroleptics) that typically reduce dopaminergic activity because too much activity has been most strongly linked to positive symptoms, specifically persecutory delusions. Dopaminergic drugs do not induce the characteristic auditory hallucinations of schizophrenia.The typical antipsychotics are known to have significant risks of side effects that can increase over time, and only show clinical effectiveness in reducing positive symptoms. Additionally, although newer atypical antipsychotics can have less affinity for dopamine receptors and still reduce positive symptoms, do not significantly reduce negative symptoms.

Psychotomimetic Glutamate Antagonists

Ketamine and PCP were observed to produce significant similarities to schizophrenia. Ketamine produces more similar symptoms (hallucinations, withdrawal) without observed permanent effects (other than ketamine tolerance). Both arylcyclohexamines have some(uM) affinity to D2 and as triple reuptake inhibitors. PCP is representative symptomatically, but does appear to cause brain structure changes seen in schizophrenia. Although unconfirmed, Dizocilpine discovered by a team at Merck seems to model both the positive and negative effects in a manner very similar to schizophreniform disorders.

Possible Glutamate Based Treatment

An early clinical trial by Eli Lilly of the drug LY2140023 has shown potential for treating schizophrenia without the weight gain and other side-effects associated with conventional anti-psychotics. A trial in 2009 failed to prove superiority over placebo or Olanzapine, but Lilly explained this as being due to an exceptionally high placebo response. However, Eli Lilly terminated further development of the compound in 2012 after it failed in phase III clinical trials. This drug acts as a selective agonist at metabotropic mGluR2 and mGluR3 glutamate receptors (the mGluR3 gene has previously been associated with schizophrenia).

Studies of glycine (and related co-agonists at the NMDA receptor) added to conventional anti-psychotics have also found some evidence that these may improve symptoms in schizophrenia.

Animal Models

Research done on mice in early 2009 has shown that when the neuregulin-1\ErbB post-synaptic receptor genes are deleted, the dendritic spines of glutamate neurons initially grow, but break down during later development. This led to symptoms (such as disturbed social function, inability to adapt to predictable future stressors) that overlap with schizophrenia. This parallels the time delay for symptoms setting in with schizophrenic humans who usually appear to show normal development until early adulthood.

Disrupted in schizophrenia 1 is a gene that is disrupted in schizophrenia.

Dopamine Hypothesis of Schizophrenia

The dopamine hypothesis of schizophrenia or the dopamine hypothesis of psychosis is a model, attributing symptoms of schizophrenia (like psychoses) to a disturbed and hyperactive dopaminergic signal transduction. The model draws evidence from the observation that a large number of antipsychotics have dopamine-receptor antagonistic effects. The theory, however, does not posit dopamine overabundance as a complete explanation for schizophrenia. Rather, the overactivation of D2 receptors, specifically, is one effect of the global chemical synaptic dysregulation observed in this disorder.

Introduction

Some researchers have suggested that dopamine systems in the mesolimbic pathway may contribute to the 'positive symptoms' of schizophrenia (whereas problems with dopamine function in the mesocortical pathway may be responsible for the 'negative symptoms', such as avolition and alogia.) Abnormal expression, thus distribution of the D_2 receptor between these areas and the rest of the brain may also be implicated in schizophrenia, specifically in the acute phase. A relative excess of these receptors within the limbic system means Broca's area, which can produce illogical language, has an abnormal connection to Wernicke's area, which comprehends language but does not create it. Note that variation in distribution is observed within individuals, so abnormalities of this characteristic likely play a significant role in all psychological illnesses. Individual alterations are produced by differences within glutamatergic pathways within the limbic system, which are also implicated in other psychotic syndromes. Among the alterations of both synaptic and global structure, the most significant abnormalities are observed in the uncinate fasciculus and the cingulate cortex. The combination of these creates a profound dissymmetry of prefrontal inhibitory signaling, shifted positively towards the dominant side. Eventually, the cingulate gyrus becomes atrophied towards the anterior, due to long-Term Depression (LTD) and Long-Term Potentiation (LTP) from the abnormally strong signals transversely across the brain. This, combined with a relative deficit in GABAergic input to Wernicke's area, shifts the balance of bilateral communication across the corpus callosum posteriorly. Through this mechanism, hemispherical communication becomes highly shifted towards the left/dominant posterior. As such, spontaneous language from Broca's can propagate through the limbic system to the tertiary auditory cortex. This retrograde signaling to the temporal lobes, results in the parietal lobes not recognizing it as internal, resulting in the auditory hallucinations typical of chronic schizophrenia.

In addition, significant cortical grey matter volume reductions are observed in this disorder. Specifically, the right hemisphere atrophies more, while both sides show a marked decrease in frontal and posterior volume. This indicates abnormal synaptic plasticity occurs, where certain feedback loops become so potentiated, others receive little glutaminergic transmission. This is a direct result of the abnormal dopaminergic input to the striatum, thus (indirectly) disinhibition of thalamic activity. The excitatory nature of dopaminergic transmission means the glutamate hypothesis of schizophrenia is inextricably intertwined with this altered functioning. 5-HT also regulates monoamine neurotransmitters, including dopaminergic transmission. Specifically, the 5-HT2A receptor regulates cortical input to the basal ganglia and many typical and atypical antipsychotics are antagonists at this receptor. Several antipsychotics are also antagonists at the 5-HT2C receptor, leading to dopamine release in the structures where 5-HT2C is expressed; striatum, prefrontal cortex, nucleus accumbens, amygdala, hippocampus (all structures indicated in this disease), and currently thought to be a reason why antipsychotics with 5HT2C antagonistic properties improves negative symptoms. More research is needed to explain the exact nature of the altered chemical transmission in this disorder.

Recent evidence on a variety of animal models of psychosis, such as sensitization of animal behaviour by amphetamine, or phencyclidine (PCP, Angel Dust), or excess steroids, or by removing various genes (COMT, DBH, GPRK6, RGS9, RIIbeta), or making brain lesions in newborn animals, or delivering animals abnormally by Caesarian section, all induce a marked behavioural supersensitivity to dopamine and a marked rise in the number of dopamine D_2 receptors in the high-affinity state for dopamine. This latter work implies that there are multiple genes and neuronal pathways that can lead to psychosis and that all these multiple psychosis pathways converge via the high-affinity state of the D2 receptor, the common target for all antipsychotics, typical or atypical. Combined with less inhibitory signalling from the thalamus and other basal ganglic structures, from hyoptrophy the abnormal activation of the cingulate cortex, specifically around Broca's and Wernicke's areas, abnormal D_2 agonism can facilitate the self-reinforcing, illogical patterns of language found in such patients. In schizophrenia, this feedback loop has progressed, which produced the widespread neural atrophy characteristic of this disease. Patients on neuroleptic or antipsychotic medication have significantly less atrophy within these crucial areas. As such, early medical intervention is crucial in preventing the advancement of these profound deficits in bilateral communication at the root of all psychotic disorders. Advanced, chronic schizophrenia can not respond even to clozapine, regarded as the most potent antipsychotic, as such, a cure for highly advanced schizophrenia is likely impossible, so the value of early intervention cannot be stressed enough.

Discussion

Evidence for the Dopamine Hypothesis

Amphetamine, cocaine and similar drugs increase levels of dopamine in the brain and can cause symptoms which resemble those present in psychosis, particularly after large doses or prolonged use. This is often referred to as "amphetamine psychosis" or "cocaine psychosis," but may produce experiences virtually indistinguishable from the positive symptoms associated with schizophrenia. Similarly, those treated with dopamine enhancing levodopa for Parkinson's disease can experience psychotic side effects mimicking the symptoms of schizophrenia. Up to 75% of patients with schizophrenia have increased signs and symptoms of their psychosis upon challenge with moderate doses of methylphenidate or amphetamine or other dopamine-like compounds, all given at doses at which control normal volunteers do not have any psychologically disturbing effects.

Some functional neuroimaging studies have also shown that, after taking amphetamine, patients diagnosed with schizophrenia show greater levels of dopamine release (particularly in the striatum) than non-psychotic individuals. However, the acute effects of dopamine stimulants include euphoria, alertness and over-confidence; these symptoms are more reminiscent of mania than schizophrenia. Since the 2000s, several PET studies have confirmed an altered synthesis capacity of dopamine in the nigrostriatal system demonstrating a dopaminergic dysregulation.

A group of drugs called the phenothiazines, including antipsychotics such as chlorpromazine, has been found to antagonize dopamine binding (particularly at receptors known as D_2 dopamine receptors) and reduce positive psychotic symptoms. This observation was subsequently extended to other antipsychotic drug classes, such as butyrophenones including haloperidol. The link was strengthened by experiments in the 1970s which suggested that the binding affinity of antipsychotic drugs for D_2 dopamine receptors seemed to be inversely proportional to their therapeutic dose. This correlation, suggesting that receptor binding is causally related to therapeutic potency, was reported by two laboratories in 1976.

Genetic evidence has suggested that there may be genes, or specific variants of genes, that code for mechanisms involved in dopamine function, which may be more prevalent in people experiencing psychosis or diagnosed with schizophrenia. Dopamine related genes linked to psychosis in this way include COMT, DRD4, and AKT1.

People with Schizophrenia appear to have a high rate of self-medication with nicotine; the therapeutic effect likely occurs through dopamine modulation by nicotinic acetylcholine receptors.

However, there was controversy and conflicting findings over whether postmortem findings resulted from drug tolerance to chronic antipsychotic treatment. Compared to the success of postmortem studies in finding profound changes of dopamine receptors, imaging studies using SPET and PET methods in drug naive patients have generally failed to find any difference in dopamine D_2 receptor density compared to controls. Comparable findings in longitudinal studies show: " Particular emphasis is given to methodological limitations in the existing literature, including lack of reliability data, clinical heterogeneity among studies, and inadequate study designs and statistic," suggestions are made for improving future longitudinal neuroimaging studies of treatment effects in schizophrenia A recent review of imaging studies in schizophrenia shows confidence in the techniques, while discussing such operator error. In 2007 one report said, "During the last decade, results of brain imaging studies by use of PET and SPET in schizophrenic patients showed a clear dysregulation of the dopaminergic system."

Recent findings from meta-analyses suggest that there may be a small elevation in dopamine D_2 receptors in drug-free patients with schizophrenia, but the degree of overlap between patients and controls makes it unlikely that this is clinically meaningful. While the review by Laruelle acknowledged more sites were found using methylspiperone, it discussed the theoretical reasons behind such an increase (including the monomer-dimer equilibrium) and called for more work to be done to 'characterise' the differences. In addition, newer antipsychotic medication (called atypical antipsychotic medication) can be as potent as older medication (called typical antipsychotic medication) while also affecting serotonin function and having somewhat less of a dopamine blocking effect. In addition, dopamine pathway dysfunction has not been reliably shown to correlate with symptom onset or severity. HVA levels correlate trendwise to symptoms severity. During the application of debrisoquin, this correlation becomes significant.

Giving a more precise explanation of this discrepancy in D_2 receptor has been attempted by a significant minority. Radioligand imaging measurements involve the monomer and dimer ratio, and the 'cooperativity' model. Cooperativitiy is a chemical function in the study of enzymes. Dopamine receptors interact with their own kind, or other receptors to form higher order receptors such as dimers, via the mechanism of cooperativity. Philip Seeman has said: "In schizophrenia, therefore, the density of [11C] methylspiperone sites rises, reflecting an increase in monomers, while the density of [11C] raclopride sites remains the same, indicating that the total population of D_2 monomers and dimers does not change." (In another place Seeman has said methylspiperone possibly binds with dimers) With this difference in measurement technique in mind, the above-mentioned meta-analysis uses results from 10 different ligands. Exaggerated ligand binding results such as SDZ GLC 756 were explained by reference to this monomer-dimer equilibrium.

According to Seeman, "...Numerous postmortem studies have consistently revealed D_2 receptors to be elevated in the striata of patients with schizophrenia". However, the authors were concerned the effect of medication may not have been fully accounted for. The study introduced an experiment by Abi-Dargham et al. in which it was shown medication-free live schizophrenics had more D_2 receptors involved in the schizophrenic process and more dopamine. Since then another study has shown such elevated percentages in D_2 receptors is brain-wide (using a different ligand, which did not need dopamine depletion). In a 2009 study, Annisa Abi-Dagham *et al.* confirmed the findings of her previous study regarding increased baseline D_2 receptors in schizophrenics and showing a correlation between this magnitude and the result of amphetamine stimulation experiments.

Some animal models of psychosis are similar to those for addiction – displaying increased locomotor activity. For those female animals with previous sexual experience, amphetamine stimulation happens faster than for virgins. There is no study on male equivalent because the studies are meant to explain why females experience addiction earlier than males.

Even in 1986 the effect of antipsychotics on receptor measurement was controversial. An article in *Science* sought to clarify whether the increase was solely due to medication by using drug-naive schizophrenics: "The finding that D_2 dopamine receptors are substantially increased in schizophrenic patients who have never been treated with neuroleptic drugs raises the possibility that dopamine receptors are involved in the schizophrenic disease process itself. Alternatively, the increased D_2 receptor number may reflect presynaptic factors such as increased endogenous dopamine levels (16). In either case, our findings support the hypothesis that dopamine receptor abnormalities are present in untreated schizophrenic patients." (The experiment used 3-N-[11C] methylspiperone – the same as mentioned by Seeman detects D_2 monomers and binding was double that of controls.)

It is still thought that dopamine mesolimbic pathways may be hyperactive, resulting in hyperstimulation of D_2 receptors and positive symptoms. There is also growing evidence that, conversely, mesocortical pathway dopamine projections to the prefrontal cortex might be hypoactive (underactive), resulting in hypostimulation of D_1 receptors, which may be related to negative symptoms and cognitive impairment. The overactivity and underactivity in these different regions may be linked, and may not be due to a primary dysfunction of dopamine systems but to more general neurodevelopmental issues that precede them. Increased dopamine sensitivity may be a common final pathway.

Another finding is a six-fold excess of binding sites insensitive to the testing agent, raclopride; Seeman said this increase was probably due to the increase in D_2 monomers. Such an increase in monomers may occur via the cooperativity mechanism which is responsible for D_2^{High} and D_2^{Low}, the supersensitive and lowsensitivity states of the D_2 dopamine receptor. More specifically, "an increase in monomers, may be one basis for dopamine supersensitivity".

Evidence Against the Dopamine Hypothesis

Further experiments, conducted as new methods were developed (particularly the ability to use PET scanning to examine drug action in the brain of living patients) challenged the view that the amount of dopamine blocking was correlated with clinical benefit. These studies showed that some patients had over 90% of their D_2 receptors blocked by antipsychotic drugs, but showed little reduction in their psychoses. This primarily occurs in patients who have had the psychosis for ten to thirty years. At least 90-95% of first-episode patients, however, respond to antipsychotics at low doses and do so with D_2 occupancy of 60-70%. The antipsychotic aripiprazole occupies over 90% of D_2 receptors, but this drug is both an agonist and an antagonist at D_2 receptors.

Furthermore, although dopamine-inhibiting medications modify dopamine levels within minutes, the associated improvement in patient symptoms is usually not visible for at least several days, suggesting that dopamine may be indirectly responsible for the illness.

Similarly, a new generation of antipsychotic drugs (called the atypical antipsychotics) were found to be just as effective as older typical antipsychotic drugs in controlling psychosis, but more effective in controlling the negative symptoms, despite the fact that they have lower affinity for dopamine receptors than for various other neurotransmitter receptors. More recent work, however, has shown that atypical antipsychotic drugs such as clozapine and quetiapine bind and unbind rapidly and repeatedly to the dopamine D_2 receptor. All of these drugs exhibit inverse agonistic effects at the $5\text{-}HT_{2A/2C}$ receptors, meaning serotonin abnormalities are also involved in the complex constellation of neurologic factors predisposing one to the self reinforcing language-based psychological deficits found in all forms of psychosis.

The excitatory neurotransmitter glutamate is now also thought to be associated with schizophrenia. Phencyclidine (also known as PCP or "Angel Dust") and ketamine, both of which block glutamate (NMDA) receptors, are known to cause psychosis at least somewhat resembling schizophrenia, further suggesting that psychosis and perhaps schizophrenia cannot fully be explained in terms of dopamine function, but may also involve other neurotransmitters.

Similarly, there is now evidence to suggest there may be a number of functional and structural anomalies in the brains of some people diagnosed with schizophrenia, such as changes in grey matter density in the frontal and temporal lobes. It appears, therefore, that there are multiple causes for psychosis and schizophrenia, including gene mutations and anatomical lesions.

Psychiatrist David Healy has argued that drug companies have inappropriately promoted the dopamine hypothesis of schizophrenia as a deliberate and calculated simplification for the benefit of drug marketing.

Relationship with Glutamate

Research has shown the importance of glutamate receptors, specifically N-methyl-D-aspartate receptors (NMDARs), in addition to dopamine in the etiology of schizophrenia. Mice with only 5% of the normal levels of NMDAR's expressed schizophrenic like behaviors seen in animal models of schizophrenia while mice with 100% of NMDAR's behaved normally. Schizophrenic behavior in low NMDAR mice has been effectively treated with antipsychotics that lower dopamine. NMDAR's and dopamine receptors in the prefrontal cortex are associated with the cognitive impairments and working memory deficits commonly seen in schizophrenia. Rats that have been given a NMDAR antagonist exhibit a significant decrease in performance on cognitive tasks. Rats given a dopamine antagonist (antipsychotic) experience a reversal of the negative effects of the NMDAR antagonist. Glutamate imbalances appear to cause abnormal functioning in dopamine. When levels of glutamate are low dopamine is overactive and results in the expression schizophrenic symptoms.

People with Schizophrenia also have a higher incidence of nicotine use than those without schizophrenia. The high rate of use may be a form of self-medication that reduces negative symptoms by increasing the activity of glutamate and lowering the activity of dopamine. Elevated activation in the prefrontal cortex from nicotine use can increase focus and cognitive performance which are impaired in people with schizophrenia. Activation of nicotinic acetylcholine receptors in mice has been shown to increase glutamate levels in the prefrontal cortex and may help to decrease the cognitive deficits seen in schizophrenia. In addition, nicotine is thought to help regulate dopamine release. Nicotine acts as an agonist to nicotinic acetylcholine receptors which then increases the release of dopamine. However, prolonged use of nicotine causes a diminished response to nicotine thus lowering dopamine levels long term. Nicotine use may be higher in people with schizophrenia because it helps to balance levels of glutamate and dopamine in the brain causing a reduction in some negative symptoms.

Criticisms

Dr Ronald Pies the current editor in Chief Emeritus of Psychiatric Times with a circulation of about 50,000 psychiatrists monthly, wrote on July 11, 2011 " In truth, the "chemical imbalance" notion was always a kind of urban legend- - never a theory seriously propounded by well-informed psychiatrists."

References

- Jones, Daniel (2003) [1917], Peter Roach, James Hartmann and Jane Setter, eds., English Pronouncing Dictionary, Cambridge: Cambridge University Press, ISBN 3-12-539683-2
- Parnas J; Jorgensen A (1989). "Pre-morbid psychopathology in schizophrenia spectrum". British Journal of Psychiatry. 155: 623–7. PMID 2611591. doi:10.1192/bjp.155.5.623
- "Medicinal treatment of psychosis/schizophrenia". www.sbu.se. Swedish Agency for Health Technology Assessment and Assessment of Social Services. 21 November 2012. Retrieved 26 June 2017
- Picchioni MM; Murray RM (July 2007). "Schizophrenia". BMJ. 335 (7610): 91–5. PMC 1914490. PMID 17626963. doi:10.1136/bmj.39227.616447.BE
- Current diagnosis & treatment psychiatry (2nd ed. ed.). New York: McGraw-Hill Medical. 2008. p. 48. ISBN 9780071422925
- Craddock N; Owen MJ (2010). "The Kraepelinian dichotomy - going, going... But still not gone". The British Journal of Psychiatry. 196: 92–95. PMC 2815936. PMID 20118450. doi:10.1192/bjp.bp.109.073429
- Cirillo, Michael; Seidman, Larry (2003). "Verbal declarative memory dysfunction in schizophrenia: from clinical assessment to genetics and brain mechanisms". Neuropsychology Review. Retrieved 14 December 2015
- Baier M (August 2010). "Insight in schizophrenia: a review". Current psychiatry reports. 12 (4): 356–61. PMID 20526897. doi:10.1007/s11920-010-0125-7
- American Psychiatric Association. Task Force on DSM-IV. (2000). Diagnostic and statistical manual of mental disorders: DSM-IV-TR. American Psychiatric Pub. ISBN 978-0-89042-025-6. p. 299
- Beck, AT (2004). "A Cognitive Model of Schizophrenia". Journal of Cognitive Psychotherapy. 18 (3): 281–88. doi:10.1891/jcop.18.3.281.65649
- "Antipsychotics for schizophrenia associated with subtle loss in brain volume". ScienceDaily. 8 February 2011. Retrieved 3 July 2014
- Kircher, Tilo & Renate Thienel (2006). "Functional brain imaging of symptoms and cognition in schizophrenia". The Boundaries of Consciousness. Amsterdam: Elsevier. p. 302. ISBN 0-444-52876-8
- Gregg L; Barrowclough C; Haddock G (2007). "Reasons for increased substance use in psychosis". Clin Psychol Rev. 27 (4): 494–510. PMID 17240501. doi:10.1016/j.cpr.2006.09.004
- Bentall RP, Read JE, Mosher LR (2004). Models of Madness: Psychological, Social and Biological Approaches to Schizophrenia. Philadelphia: Brunner-Routledge. ISBN 1-58391-906-6
- "Psychosis and schizophrenia in adults: treatment and management" (PDF). NICE. Mar 2014. p. 7. Archived from the original (PDF) on 20 April 2014. Retrieved 19 April 2014
- Kumra S; Shaw M; Merka P; Nakayama E; Augustin R (2001). "Childhood-onset schizophrenia: research update". Canadian Journal of Psychiatry. 46 (10): 923–30. PMID 11816313

- World Health Organization (2008). The global burden of disease : 2004 update ([Online-Ausg.] ed.). Geneva, Switzerland: World Health Organization. p. 35. ISBN 9789241563710
- Yuhas, Daisy. "Throughout History, Defining Schizophrenia Has Remained a Challenge (Timeline)". Scientific American Mind (March 2013). Retrieved 1 March 2013
- Pope HG (1983). "Distinguishing bipolar disorder from schizophrenia in clinical practice: guidelines and case reports". Hospital and Community Psychiatry. 34: 322–28. PMID 6840720. doi:10.1176/ps.34.4.322
- Green MF (2006). "Cognitive impairment and functional outcome in schizophrenia and bipolar disorder". Journal of Clinical Psychiatry. 67 (Suppl 9): 3–8. PMID 16965182. doi:10.4088/jcp.1006e12

6

Schizophrenia: Symptoms, Diagnosis and Management

Schizophrenia is a debilitating mental disorder that causes a variety of symptoms and complications. It is necessary to understand the basic symptoms of schizophrenia so as to assess the development of psychosis in the patient. In order to completely understand schizophrenia, it is necessary to understand the processes related to it. The following chapter elucidates the varied processes and mechanisms associated with this area of study.

Basic Symptoms of Schizophrenia

Basic symptoms of schizophrenia are subjective symptoms, described as experienced from a person's perspective, which show evidence of underlying psychopathology. Basic symptoms have generally been applied to the assessment of people who may be at risk to develop psychosis. Though basic symptoms are often disturbing for the person, problems generally do not become evident to others until the person is no longer able to cope with their basic symptoms. In the prodrome to psychosis, uncharacteristic basic symptoms develop first, followed by more characteristic basic symptoms and brief and self-limited psychotic-like symptoms, and finally the onset of psychosis. In 2015, the European Psychiatric Association issued guidance recommending the use of a subscale of basic symptoms, called the Cognitive Disturbances scale (COGDIS), in the assessment of psychosis risk in help-seeking psychiatric patients; in a meta-analysis, COGDIS was shown to be as predictive of transition to psychosis as the Ultra High Risk (UHR) criteria up to 2 years after assessment, and significantly more predictive thereafter. The basic symptoms measured by COGDIS, as well as those measured by another subscale, the Cognitive-Perceptive basic symptoms scale (COPER), are predictive of transition to schizophrenia.

Course

Basic symptoms often appear several years before the onset of psychosis, but are often preceded by the onset of self-disorders. They may sometimes appear and then disappear before appearing again much later, where they occur as part of an *outpost syndrome*. At one point, uncharacteristic basic symptoms will appear, which comprise various disturbances of mood, emotions, drive, thought, and attention that can occur in many other disorders, followed by the characteristic basic symptoms, which comprise disturbances of thought, perception, and attention, along with minor reality distortion, that are associated with schizophrenia in particular. Afterward, attenuated symptoms of psychosis or brief periods of psychosis will appear, before culminating in the emergence of full-blown psychosis. At any stage before psychosis, the person will attempt to cope with the basic symptoms, which might conceal the problems from others; once the person reaches the limit of their ability to compensate, however, the problems will become evident to others and cause impairment.

After the resolution of psychosis, basic symptoms may follow one of 3 courses: Psychosis and the basic symptoms may resolve completely allowing the restoration of normal functioning; they may remit but remain at an uncharacteristic level, with relapses of psychosis; or the characteristic basic symptoms may remain creating a deficit syndrome dominated by negative symptoms.

Evaluation

Basic symptoms are generally evaluated using the Schizophrenia Proneness Instrument (SPI), of which there are both a child and youth version (SPI-CY) and an adult version (SPI-A); this instrument assesses basic symptoms, both those that are uncharacteristic and those characteristic of psychosis. Out of the items evaluated on the SPI-CY and the SPI-A, there can be derived 2 scales to evaluate specifically the characteristic basic symptoms: the Cognitive Disturbances scale (COGDIS) and the Cognitive-Perceptual Basic Symptoms scale (COPER).

COGDIS criteria are met when at least 2 of the symptoms on the scale are present with at least weekly occurrence in the last 3 months, and which were not present during the pre-morbid phase of the illness and do not result from drug use. The European Psychiatric Association recommends the use of this scale, along with attenuated psychotic symptoms and brief transient psychosis, to detect at-risk mental states in help-seeking people.

COPER criteria are met when at least 1 of the symptoms on the scale is present with at least weekly occurrence in the last 3 months, and the first occurrence of symptoms was more than 12 months prior to evaluation.

Below are the basic symptoms associated with psychosis, along with whether they appear on COGDIS, COPER, or both:

Symptom	COGDIS	COPER	Description
Thought interference	Yes	Yes	Interference of unimportant, irrelevant thoughts that hinders thinking and concentration.
Thought perseveration	No	Yes	Repetition of thoughts that have little or no salience.
Thought pressure	Yes	Yes	Many thoughts with no common theme pop up uncontrollably.

Thought blockages	Yes	Yes	Sudden loss of train of thought that may be accompanied by the intrusion of a new thought.
Disturbance of receptive language	Yes	Yes	Lack of immediate comprehension of speech or text in one's native language.
Disturbance of expressive language	Yes	No	Difficulty producing speech or text that is appropriate to one's message in one's native language.
Disturbances of abstract thinking	Yes	No	Difficulty comprehending idioms and metaphors.
Inability to divide attention	Yes	No	Difficulty doing something with one sense (such as vision) while simultaneously using another sense for something else (such as hearing).
Captivation of attention by details of the visual field	Yes	No	Attention is drawn to unimportant details as if one were "spellbound".
Decreased ability to discriminate between perception and ideas, true memories and fantasies	No	Yes	Difficulty discriminating between what one has observed and what one has imagined.
Unstable ideas of reference with insight	Yes	Yes	Sub-psychotic referential ideation that is thereafter immediately corrected by the person.
Derealization	No	Yes	Sense of disconnect or unreality in one's environment.
Visual or acoustic perceptual disturbances with insight	No	Yes	Disturbances of the perception of brightness or loudness, color or sound quality, or distortions in one's perceptions that are recognized by the person as false.

Dual Diagnosis

Dual diagnosis (also called co-occurring disorders, COD) is the condition of suffering from a mental illness and a comorbid substance abuse problem. There is considerable debate surrounding the appropriateness of using a single category for a heterogeneous group of individuals with complex needs and a varied range of problems. The concept can be used broadly, for example depression and alcoholism, or it can be restricted to specify severe mental illness (e.g. psychosis, schizophrenia) and substance misuse disorder (e.g. cannabis abuse), or a person who has a milder mental illness and a drug dependency, such as panic disorder or generalized anxiety disorder and is dependent on opioids. Diagnosing a primary psychiatric illness in substance abusers is challenging as drug abuse itself often induces psychiatric symptoms, thus making it necessary to differentiate between substance induced and pre-existing mental illness.

Those with co-occurring disorders face complex challenges. They have increased rates of relapse, hospitalization, homelessness, and HIV and hepatitis C infection compared to those with either mental or substance use disorders alone. The cause of co-occurring disorders is unknown, although there are several theories.

Differentiating Pre-existing and Substance Induced

Drug abuse, including alcohol and prescription drugs, can induce symptomatology which resembles mental illness, which can make it difficult to differentiate between substance induced psychiatric syndromes and pre-existing mental health problems. More often than not psychiatric disorders among drug or alcohol abusers disappear with prolonged abstinence. Substance induced psychiatric symptoms can occur both in the intoxicated state and also during the withdrawal state. In some cases these substance induced psychiatric disorders can persist long after detoxification, such as prolonged psychosis or depression after amphetamine or cocaine abuse. Abuse of hallucinogens can trigger delusional and other psychotic phenomena long after cessation of use and cannabis may trigger panic attacks during intoxication and with use it may cause a state similar to dysthymia. Severe anxiety and depression are commonly induced by sustained alcohol abuse which in most cases abates with prolonged abstinence. Even moderate sustained use of alcohol may increase anxiety and depression levels in some individuals. In most cases these drug induced psychiatric disorders fade away with prolonged abstinence. A protracted withdrawal syndrome can also occur with psychiatric and other symptoms persisting for months after cessation of use. Benzodiazepines are the most notable drug for inducing prolonged withdrawal effects with symptoms sometimes persisting for years after cessation of use.

Prevalence

The 2011 USA National Survey on Drug Use and Health found that 17.5% of adults with a mental illness had a co-occurring substance use disorder; this works out to 7.98 million people. Estimates of co-occurring disorders in Canada are even higher, with an estimated 40-60% of adults with a severe and persistent mental illness experiencing a substance use disorder in their lifetime.

A study by Kessler et al. in the United States attempting to assess the prevalence of dual diagnosis found that 47% of clients with schizophrenia had a substance misuse disorder at some time in their life, and the chances of developing a substance misuse disorder was significantly higher among patients suffering from a psychotic illness than in those without a psychotic illness.

Another study looked at the extent of substance misuse in a group of 187 chronically mentally ill patients living in the community. According to the clinician's ratings, around a third of the sample used alcohol, street drugs, or both during the six months before evaluation.

Further UK studies have shown slightly more moderate rates of substance misuse among mentally ill individuals. One study found that individuals suffering from schizophrenia showed just a 7% prevalence of problematic drug use in the year prior to being interviewed and 21% reported problematic use some time before that.

Wright and colleagues identified individuals with psychotic illnesses who had been in contact with services in the London borough of Croydon over the previous 6 months. Cases of alcohol or substance misuse and dependence were identified through standardized interviews with clients and keyworkers. Results showed that prevalence rates of dual diagnosis were 33% for the use of any substance, 20% for alcohol misuse only and 5% for drug misuse only. A lifetime history of any illicit drug use was observed in 35% of the sample.

Diagnosis

Substance use disorders can be confused with other psychiatric disorders. There are diagnoses for substance-induced mood disorders and substance-induced anxiety disorders and thus such overlap can be complicated. For this reason, the DSM-IV advises that diagnoses of primary psychiatric disorders not be made in the absence of sobriety (of duration sufficient to allow for any substance-induced post-acute-withdrawal symptoms to dissipate) up to 1 year.

Treatment

Only a small proportion of those with co-occurring disorders actually receive treatment for both disorders. In 2011, it was estimated that only 12.4% of American adults with co-occurring disorders were receiving both mental health and addictions treatment. Clients with co-occurring disorders face challenges accessing treatment, as they may be excluded from mental health services if they admit to a substance abuse problem, and vice versa.

There are multiple approaches to treating concurrent disorders. Partial treatment involves treating only the disorder that is considered primary. Sequential treatment involves treating the primary disorder first, and then treating the secondary disorder after the primary disorder has been stabilized. Parallel treatment involves the client receiving mental health services from one provider, and addictions services from another.

Integrated treatment involves a seamless blending of interventions into a single coherent treatment package developed with a consistent philosophy and approach among care providers. With this approach, both disorders are considered primary. Integrated treatment can improve accessibility, service individualization, engagement in treatment, treatment compliance, mental health symptoms, and overall outcomes. The Substance Abuse and Mental Health Services Administration in the United States describes integrated treatment as being in the best interests or clients, programs, funders, and systems. Green suggested that treatment should be integrated, and a collaborative process between the treatment team and the patient. Furthermore, recovery should to be viewed as a marathon rather than a sprint, and methods and outcome goals should be explicit.

Although many patients may reject medications as antithetical to substance-abuse recovery and side effects, they can be useful to reduce paranoia, anxiety, and craving. Medications that have proven effective include opioid replacement therapies, such as lifelong maintenance on methadone or buprenorphine, to minimize risk of relapse, fatality, and legal trouble amongst opioid addicts, as well as helping with cravings, baclofen for alcoholics, opioid addicts, cocaine addicts, and amphetamine addicts, to help eliminate drug cravings, and clozapine, the first atypical antipsychotic, which appears to reduce illicit drug use amongst stimulant addicts. Clozapine can cause respiratory arrest when combined with alcohol, benzodiazepines, or opioids, so it is not recommended to use in these groups.

Theories of Dual Diagnosis

There are a number of theories that explain the relationship between mental illness and substance abuse.

Causality

The causality theory suggests that certain types of substance abuse may causally lead to mental illness.

There is strong evidence that using cannabis can produce temporary and usually mild psychotic and affective experiences. When it comes to persisting effects, there is a clear increase in incidence of psychotic outcomes in people who had used cannabis, even when they had used it only once. More frequent use of cannabis strongly augmented the risk for psychosis. The evidence for affective outcomes is less strong. However, this connection between cannabis and psychosis does not prove that cannabis *causes* psychotic disorders. The causality theory for cannabis has been challenged as despite explosive increases in cannabis consumption over the past 40 years in western society, the rate of schizophrenia (and psychosis in general) has remained relatively stable.

Attention-deficit Hyperactivity Disorder

One in four people who have a substance use disorder also have attention-deficit hyperactivity disorder, which makes the treatment of both conditions more difficult. ADHD is associated with an increased craving for drugs. Having ADHD makes it more likely that an individual will initiate substance misuse at a younger age than their peers. They are also more likely to have a poorer outcome, such as longer time to remission, and increased psychiatric complications from substance misuse. While generally stimulant medications do not seem to worsen substance misuse, they are known to be abused in some cases. Psychosocial therapy and/or nonstimulant medications and extended release stimulants are ADHD treatment options that reduce these risks.

Autism Spectrum Disorder

Unlike ADHD, which significantly increases the risk of substance use disorder, autism spectrum disorder has the opposite effect of significantly reducing the risk of substance abuse. This is because introversion, inhibition and lack of sensation seeking personality traits, which are typical of autism spectrum disorder, protect against substance abuse and thus substance abuse levels are low in individuals who are on the autism spectrum. However, certain forms of substance abuse, especially alcohol abuse, can cause or worsen certain neuropsychological symptoms which are common to autism spectrum disorder, such as impaired social skills due to the neurotoxic effects of alcohol on the brain, especially the prefrontal cortex area of the brain. The social skills that are impaired by alcohol abuse include impairments in perceiving facial emotions, prosody perception problems and theory of mind deficits; the ability to understand humour is also impaired in alcohol abusers.

Past Exposure to Psychiatric Medications Theory

The past exposure theory suggests that exposure to psychiatric medication alters neural synapses, introducing an imbalance that was not previously present. Discontinuation of the drug is expected to result in symptoms of psychiatric illness which resolve once the drug is restarted. This theory suggests that while it may appear that the medication is working, it is only treating a disorder caused by the medication itself. New exposure to psychiatric medication may lead to heightened sensitivity to the effects of drugs and alcohol, which has a deteriorating effect on the patient.

Self-medication Theory

The self-medication theory suggests that people with severe mental illnesses misuse substances in order to relieve a specific set of symptoms and counter the negative side-effects of antipsychotic medication.

Khantizan proposes that substances are not randomly chosen, but are specifically selected for their effects. For example, using stimulants such as nicotine or amphetamines can be used to combat the sedation that can be caused by higher doses of certain types of (usually typical) antipsychotic medication. Conversely, some people taking medications with a stimulant effect such as the SNRI antidepressants Effexor (venlafaxine) or Wellbutrin (bupropion) may seek out benzodiazepines or opioid narcotics to counter the anxiety and insomnia that such medications sometimes evoke.

Some studies show that nicotine administration can be effective for reducing motor side-effects of antipsychotics, with both bradykinesia (stiff muscles) and dyskinesia(involuntary movement) being prevented.

Alleviation of Dysphoria Theory

The alleviation of dysphoria theory suggests that people with severe mental illness commonly have a negative self-image, which makes them vulnerable to using psychoactive substances to alleviate these feelings. Despite the existence of a wide range of dysphoric feelings (anxiety, depression, boredom, and loneliness), the literature on self-reported reasons for use seems to lend support for the experience of these feelings being the primary motivator for drug and alcohol misuse.

Multiple Risk Factor Theory

Another theory is that there may be shared risk factors that can lead to both substance abuse and mental illness. Mueser hypothesizes that these may include factors such as social isolation, poverty, lack of structured daily activity, lack of adult role responsibility, living in areas with high drug availability, and association with people who already misuse drugs.

Other evidence suggests that traumatic life events, such as sexual abuse, are associated with the development of psychiatric problems and substance abuse.

The Supersensitivity Theory

The supersensitivity theory proposes that certain individuals who have severe mental illness also have biological and psychological vulnerabilities, caused by genetic and early environmental life events. These interact with stressful life events and can result in either a psychiatric disorder or trigger a relapse into an existing illness. The theory states that although anti-psychotic medication can reduce the vulnerability, substance abuse may increase it, causing the individual to be more likely to experience negative consequences from using relatively small amounts of substances. These individuals, therefore, are "supersensitive" to the effects of certain substances, and individuals with psychotic illness such as schizophrenia may be less capable of sustaining moderate substance use over time without experiencing negative symptoms.

Although there are limitations in the research studies conducted in this area, namely that most have focused primarily on schizophrenia, this theory provides an explanation of why relatively low levels of substance misuse often result in negative consequences for individuals with severe mental illness.

History

The traditional method for treating patients suffering from dual diagnosis was a parallel treatment program. In this format, patients received mental health services from one clinician while addressing their substance abuse with a separate clinician. However, researchers found that parallel treatments were ineffective, suggesting a need to integrate the services addressing mental health with those addressing substance abuse.

During the mid-1980s, a number of initiatives began to combine mental health and substance abuse services in an attempt to meet this need. These programs worked to shift the method of treatment for substance abuse from a confrontational approach to a supportive one. They also introduced new methods to motivate clients and worked with them to develop long-term goals for their care. Although the studies conducted by these initiatives did not have control groups, their results were promising and became the basis for more rigorous efforts to study and develop models of integrated treatment.

Stimulant Psychosis

Stimulant psychosis is a psychosis symptom which typically occurs following an overdose on psychostimulants, but it also occurs in approximately 0.1% of individuals within the first several weeks after starting amphetamine or methylphenidate therapy.

The most common causative agents are substituted amphetamines and cocaine.

Signs and Symptoms

The symptoms of stimulant psychosis may vary slightly depending on the drug ingested but generally include the symptoms of organic psychosis including hallucinations, delusions, and thought disorder.

Stimulants Known to Cause Psychosis

Substituted Amphetamines

Drugs in the class of amphetamines, or substituted amphetamines, are known to induce "amphetamine psychosis" typically when chronically abused or used in high doses. In an Australian study of 309 active methamphetamine users, 18% had experienced a clinical level psychosis in the past year. Common amphetamines include cathinone, DOM, ephedrine, MDMA, methamphetamine, and methcathinone though a large number of such compounds have been synthesized. Methylphenidate is sometimes incorrectly included in this class.

The symptoms of amphetamine psychosis include auditory and visual hallucinations, delusions of persecution, and delusions of reference concurrent with both clear consciousness and prominent extreme agitation. A Japanese study of recovery from methamphetamine psychosis reported a 64% recovery rate within 10 days rising to an 82% recovery rate at 30 days after methamphetamine cessation. However it has been suggested that around 5–15% of users fail to make a complete recovery in the long term. Furthermore, even at a small dose, the psychosis can be quickly reestablished. Psychosocial stress has been found to be an independent risk factor for psychosis relapse even without further substituted amphetamine use in certain cases.

The symptoms of acute amphetamine psychosis are very similar to those of the acute phase of schizophrenia although in amphetamine psychosis visual hallucinations are more common and thought disorder is rare. Amphetamine psychosis may be purely related to high drug usage, or high drug usage may trigger an underlying vulnerability to schizophrenia. There is some evidence that vulnerability to amphetamine psychosis and schizophrenia may be genetically related. Relatives of methamphetamine users with a history of amphetamine psychosis are five times more likely to have been diagnosed with schizophrenia than relatives of methamphetamine users without a history of amphetamine psychosis. The disorders are often distinguished by a rapid resolution of symptoms in amphetamine psychosis, while schizophrenia is more likely to follow a chronic course.

Although rare and not formally recognized, a condition known as Amphetamine Withdrawal Psychosis (AWP) may occur upon cessation of substituted amphetamine use and, as the name implies, involves psychosis that appears on withdrawal from substituted amphetamines. However, unlike similar disorders, in AWP, substituted amphetamines reduce rather than increase symptoms, and the psychosis or mania resolves with resumption of the previous dosing schedule.

Cocaine

Cocaine has a similar potential to induce temporary psychosis with more than half of cocaine abusers reporting at least some psychotic symptoms at some point. Typical symptoms of sufferers include paranoid delusions that they are being followed and that their drug use is being watched, accompanied by hallucinations that support the delusional beliefs. Delusional parasitosis with formication ("cocaine bugs") is also a fairly common symptom.

Cocaine-induced psychosis shows sensitization toward the psychotic effects of the drug. This means that psychosis becomes more severe with repeated intermittent use.

Methylphenidate

Chronic abuse of methylphenidate can also lead to psychosis. Psychotic symptoms from methylphenidate can include hearing voices, visual hallucinations, urges to harm oneself, severe anxiety, mania, grandiosity, paranoid delusions, confusion, increased aggression, and irritability.

Caffeine

There is limited evidence that caffeine, in high doses or when chronically abused, may induce psychosis in normal individuals and worsen pre-existing psychosis in those diagnosed with schizophrenia.

Treatment

Treatment consists of supportive care during the acute intoxication phase: maintaining hydration, body temperature, blood pressure, and heart rate at acceptable levels until the drug is sufficiently metabolized to allow vital signs to return to baseline. Typical and atypical antipsychotics have been shown to be helpful in the early stages of treatment. This is followed by abstinence from psychostimulants supported with counseling or medication designed to assist the individual preventing a relapse and the resumption of a psychotic state.

Distinction from Excited Delirium

Though less common than stimulant psychosis, stimulants such as cocaine and amphetamines as well as the dissociative drug phencyclidine (PCP, angel dust) may also cause a theorized severe and life-threatening condition known as excited delirium. This condition manifests as a combination of delirium, psychomotor agitation, anxiety, delusions, hallucinations, speech disturbances, disorientation, violent and bizarre behavior, insensitivity to pain, elevated body temperature, and superhuman strength. Despite some superficial similarities in presentation excited delirium is a distinct (and more serious) condition than stimulant psychosis. The existence of excited delirium is currently debated.

Self-disorder

A self-disorder, also called ipseity disturbance, is a psychological phenomenon of disruption or diminishing of a person's sense of minimal (or basic) self. The sense of minimal self refers to the very basic sense of having experiences that are one's own; it has no properties, unlike the more extended sense of self, the narrative self, which is characterized by the person's reflections on themselves as a person, things they like, their identity, and other aspects that are the result of reflection on one's self. Disturbances in the sense of minimal self, as measured by the Examination of Anomalous Self-Experience (EASE), aggregate in the schizophrenia spectrum disorders, to include schizotypal personality disorder, and distinguish them from other conditions such as psychotic bipolar disorder and borderline personality disorder.

Minimal Self

The minimal self has been likened to a "flame that enlightens its surroundings and thereby itself." Unlike the extended self, which is composed of properties such as the person's identity, the person's narrative, and other aspects that can be gleaned from reflection, the minimal self has no properties, but refers to the "mine-ness" "given-ness" of experience, that the experiences are that of the person having them in that person's stream of consciousness. These experiences that are part of the minimal self are normally "tacit" and implied, requiring no reflection on the part of the person experiencing to know that the experience is theirs. The minimal self cannot be further elaborated and normally one cannot grasp it upon reflection. The minimal self goes hand-in-hand with immersion in the shared social world, such that "[t]he world is always pregiven, ie, tacitly grasped as a self-evident background of all experiencing and meaning." This is the self-world structure.

De Warren gives an example of the minimal self combined with immersion in the shared social world: "When looking at this tree in my backyard, my consciousness is directed toward the tree and not toward my own act of perception. I am, however, aware of myself as perceiving this tree, yet this self-awareness (or self-consciousness) is not itself thematic." The focus is normally on the tree itself, not on the person's own act of seeing the tree: to know that one is seeing the tree does not require an act of reflection.

Disturbance

In the schizophrenia spectrum disorders, the minimal self and the self-world structure are "constantly *challenged, unstable,* and *oscillating,*" causing anomalous self-experiences known as self-disorders. These involve the person feeling as if they lack an identity, as if they are not really existing, that the sense of their experiences being their own (the "mine-ness" of their experiential world) is failing or diminishing, as if their inner experiences are no longer private, and that they don't really understand the world. These experiences lead to the person engaging in *hyper-reflectivity*, or abnormally prolonged and intense self-reflection, to attempt to gain a grasp on these experiences, but such intense reflection may further exacerbate the self-disorders. Self-disorders tend to be chronic, becoming incorporated into the person's way of being and affecting "how" they experience the world and not necessarily "what" they experience. This instability of the minimal self may provoke the onset of psychosis.

Similar phenomena can occur in other conditions, such as bipolar disorder and depersonalization disorder, but Sass's (2014) review of the literature comparing accounts of self-experience in various mental disorders shows that serious self-other confusion and "severe erosion of minimal self-experience" only occur in schizophrenia; as an example of the latter, Sass cites the autobiographical account of Elyn Saks, who has schizophrenia, of her experience of "disorganization" in which she felt that thoughts, perceptions, sensations, and even the passage of time became incoherent, and that she had no longer "the solid center from which one experiences reality", which occurred when she was 7 or 8 years old. This disturbance tends to fluctuate over time based on emotions and motivation, accounting for the phenomenon of *dialipsis* in schizophrenia, where neurocognitive performance tends to be inconsistent over time.

The disturbance of the minimal self may manifest in people in various ways, including as a tendency to inspect one's thoughts in order to know what they are thinking, like a person seeing an image, reading a message, or listening closely to someone talking. In normal thought, the "signifier" (the images or inner speech representing the thought) and the "meaning" are combined into the "expression", so that the person "inhabits" their thinking, or that both the signifier and the meaning implicitly come to mind together; the person does not need to reflect on their thoughts to understand what they are thinking. In people with self-disorder, however, it is frequently the case that many thoughts are experienced as more like external objects that are not implicitly comprehended. The person must turn their focus toward the thoughts to understand their thoughts because of that lack of implicit comprehension, a split of the signifier and the meaning from each other, where the signifier emerges automatically in the field of awareness but the meaning does not. This is an example of the failing "mine-ness" of the experiential field as the minimal self recedes from its own thoughts, which are consigned to an outer space. This is present chronically, both during and outside of psychosis, and may represent a middle point between normal inner speech and auditory hallucinations, as well as normal experience and first-rank symptoms.

They may also experience uncontrolled multiple trains of thought with different themes simultaneously coursing through one's head interfering with concentration (*thought pressure*) or often feel they must attend to things with their full attention in order to get done what most people can do without giving it much thought (*hyper-reflectivity*), which can lead to fatigue.

Clinical Relevance

The presence of self-disorders may have predictive power for whether those with an at risk mental state will develop psychosis; the risk of suicidal ideation and suicide by people with schizophrenia, though depression would also be an important factor; predicting initial social dysfunction in people with either schizophrenic or bipolar psychosis; and whether a person will move to a schizophrenia spectrum diagnosis later.

The presence of self-disorders may cause reduced person insight into their illness through the alteration of the basic structures of consciousness.

Self-disorders are difficult for the people experiencing them to articulate spontaneously; and are not well-known, by either the general public or professionals in the field. Because of this, people will often make vague, cliched complaints that mimic the symptoms of other mental disorders, symptoms such as "fatigue" or "concentration difficulties". Were a knowledgeable clinician to probe deeper, however, the underlying self-disorders may be assessed and help clarify the nature of the person's illness. In their review, Parnas, et al. (2014) say, "The psychiatrist's acquaintance with the phenomenon of 'non-specific specificity' is, in our view, extremely important in the context of early diagnostic assessment, especially of people presenting with a vague, unelaborated picture of maladjustment, underperformance, chronic malaise and dysphoria, negative symptoms, or hypochondriac preoccupations." People with schizophrenia often describe their self-disorders as causing more suffering for them than psychosis.

Self-disorders underlie most of the first-rank symptoms, those often termed passivity phenomena. There is a current proposal to list self-disorder as one of the symptoms of schizophrenia in the upcoming ICD-11.

Future Directions and Controversy

In a 2014 review, Postmes, et al., suggested that self-disorders and psychosis may arise from attempts to compensate for perceptual incoherence and proposed a hypothesis for how the interaction among these phenomena and the person's attempts to resolve the incoherence give rise to schizophrenia. The problems with the integration of sensory information create problems for the person in keeping a grip on the world, and since the self-world interaction is fundamentally linked to the basic sense of self, the latter is also disrupted as a result. Sass and Borda have studied the correlates of the dimensions of self-disorders, namely *disturbed grip* (perplexity, difficulty "getting" stuff most people can get), *hyperreflexivity* (where thoughts, feelings, sensations, and objects pop up uncontrollably in the field of awareness, as well dysfunctional reflecting on matters and the self), and *diminished self-affection* (where the person has difficulty being "affected" by aspects of the self, experiencing those aspects as if they existed in an outer space), and have proposed how both primary and secondary factors may arise from dysfunctions in perceptual organization and multisensory integration.

In a 2013 review, Mishara, et al., criticized the concept of the minimal self as an explanation for self-disorder, saying that it is unfalsifiable, and that self-disorder arises primarily from difficulty integrating different aspects of the self as well as having difficulty distinguishing self and other, as proposed by Lysaker and Lysaker: *Ichstörung* or ego disorder, as they say, in schizophrenia arises from disturbed relationships not from the "solipsistic" concept of the self as proposed by Sass, Parnas, and others. In his review, Sass agrees that the focus of research into self-disorder has focused too much on the self, and mentions attempts to look at disturbances in the person's relationship with other people and the world, with work being done to create an Examination of Anomalous World Experience, which will look at the person's anomalous experiences regarding time, space, persons, language, and atmosphere; he suggests there are problems with both the self and the world in people with self-disorder, and that it may be better conceptualized as a "presence-disturbance". Parnas acknowledges the Lysaker model, but says that it is not incompatible with the concept of the minimal self, as they deal with different levels of self-hood.

History of the Concept

The concept of a basic self-disturbance in schizophrenia appears in all the foundational texts on the disease. However, the concept was difficult to operationalize and was criticized for being vague and too subjective; little systematic or empirical research was done on the concept in the 20th century. The publication of the DSM-III (1980) had unintended consequences, however, and led, in many instances, to focusing only on the signs and symptoms listed as criteria and generally ignoring the other signs and symptoms that can appear with each disorder; it privileged a behaviorist approach to diagnosis. The concept of this self-disturbance soon disappeared from training programs in the United States.

The Bonn Scale for the Assessment of Basic Symptoms was created to assess sub-clinical affective, cognitive and perceptual disturbances, as well as basic self-disturbance, in people, and in many studies basic symptoms were found to aggregate in people with schizophrenic and schizotypal disorders. Basic symptoms are subjective and difficult for the person to describe spontaneously, but the person will try to adapt and cope with them: functioning becomes impaired when people reach their adaptive capacity. In the period leading up to the first episode of schizophrenia, uncharacteristic basic symptoms first appear and are followed by the onset of more characteristic basic symptoms and, finally, psychosis.

To revive the concept of basic self-disturbance and to overcome the previous problems of a lack of a concrete definition of it, a group of researchers developed the EASE, based on phenomenological interviews with first-admission people with schizophrenia spectrum disorders, to enable empirical research of self-disorders.

Thought Disorder

Thought disorder (TD) or formal thought disorder (FTD) refers to disorganized thinking as evidenced by disorganized speech. Specific thought disorders include derailment, poverty of speech, tangentiality, illogicality, perseveration, and thought blocking.

Psychiatrists consider formal thought disorder as being one of two types of disordered thinking, with the other type being delusions. The latter involves "content" while the former involves "form". Although the term "thought disorder" can refer to either type, in common parlance it refers most often to a disorder of thought "form" also known as formal thought disorder.

Eugen Bleuler, who named schizophrenia, held that thought disorder was its defining characteristic. However, formal thought disorder is not unique to schizophrenia or psychosis. It is often a symptom of mania, and less often it can be present in other mental disorders such as depression. Clanging or echolalia may be present in Tourette syndrome. Patients with a clouded consciousness, like that found in delirium, also have a formal thought disorder.

However, there is a clinical difference between these two groups. Those with schizophrenia or psychosis are less likely to demonstrate awareness or concern about the disordered thinking. Clayton and Winokur have suggested that this results from a fundamental inability to use the same type of Aristotelian logic as others. On the other hand, patients with a clouded consciousness, referred to as "organic" patients, usually do demonstrate awareness and concern, and complain about being "confused" or "unable to think straight"; Clayton and Winokur suggest that this is because their thought disorder results, instead, from various cognitive deficits.

Signs and Symptoms

In considering whether an individual has thought disorder, patterns of their speech are closely observed. Although it is normal to exhibit some of the following during times of extreme stress (e.g. a cataclysmic event or the middle of a war) it is the degree, frequency, and the resulting functional impairment that leads to the conclusion that the person being observed has a thought disorder.

- *Alogia* (also *poverty of speech*) – A poverty of speech, either in amount or content; it can occur as a negative symptom of schizophrenia.
- *Blocking* – An abrupt stop in the middle of a train of thought; the individual may or may not be able to continue the idea. This is a type of formal thought disorder that can be seen in schizophrenia.
- *Circumstantiality* (also *circumstantial thinking*, or *circumstantial speech*) – An inability to answer a question without giving excessive, unnecessary detail. This differs from tangential thinking, in that the person does eventually return to the original point.
- *Clanging* or *Clang association* – a severe form of flight of ideas whereby ideas are related only by similar or rhyming sounds rather than actual meaning. This may be heard as excessive rhyming and/or alliteration. e.g. "Many moldy mushrooms merge out of the mildewy mud on Mondays." "I heard the bell. Well, hell, then I fell." It is most commonly seen in bipolar affective disorder (manic phase), although it is often observed in patients with primary psychoses, namely schizophrenia and schizoaffective disorder.
- *Derailment* (also *loose association* and *knight's move thinking*) – Thought and/or speech move, either spontaneously or in response to an internal stimulus (distinguishing derailment from "distractible speech," *infra*), from the topic's track onto another which is obliquely related or unrelated. e.g. "The next day when I'd be going out you know, I took control, like uh, I put bleach on my hair in California."
- *Distractible speech* – During mid speech, the subject is changed in response to an external stimulus. e.g. "Then I left San Francisco and moved to... where did you get that tie?"
- *Echolalia* – Echoing of another's speech that may only be committed once, or may be continuous in repetition. This may involve repeating only the last few

words or last word of the examiner's sentences. This can be a symptom of Tourette's Syndrome. e.g. "What would you like for dinner?", "That's a good question. *That's a good question. That's a good question. That's a good question.*"

- *Evasive interaction* – Attempts to express ideas and/or feelings about another individual come out as evasive or in a diluted form, e.g.: "I... er ah... you are uh... I think you have... uh-- acceptable erm... uh... hair."
- "Flight of ideas" – a form of formal thought disorder marked by abrupt leaps from one topic to another, albeit with discernable links between successive ideas, perhaps governed by similarities between subjects or, in somewhat higher grades, by rhyming, puns, and word plays (clang associations), or innocuous environmental stimuli – e.g., the sound of birds chirping. It is most characteristic of the manic phase of bipolar illness.
- *Illogicality* – Conclusions are reached that do not follow logically (non-sequiturs or faulty inferences). e.g. "Do you think this will fit in the box?" draws a reply like "Well duh; it's brown, isn't it?"
- *Incoherence (word salad)* – Speech that is unintelligible because, though the individual words are real words, the manner in which they are strung together results in incoherent gibberish, e.g. the question "Why do people comb their hair?" elicits a response like "Because it makes a twirl in life, my box is broken help me blue elephant. Isn't lettuce brave? I like electrons, hello please!"
- *Loss of goal* – Failure to follow a train of thought to a natural conclusion. e.g. "Why does my computer keep crashing?", "Well, you live in a stucco house, so the pair of scissors needs to be in another drawer."
- *Neologisms* – New word formations. These may also involve elisions of two words that are similar in meaning or in sound. e.g. "I got so angry I picked up a dish and threw it at the geshinker."
- *Perseveration* – Persistent repetition of words or ideas even when another person attempts to change the topic. e.g. "It's great to be here in Nevada, Nevada, Nevada, Nevada, Nevada." This may also involve repeatedly giving the same answer to different questions. e.g. "Is your name Mary?" "Yes." "Are you in the hospital?" "Yes." "Are you a table?" "Yes." Perseveration can include palilalia and logoclonia, and can be an indication of organic brain disease such as Parkinson's.
- *Phonemic paraphasia* – Mispronunciation; syllables out of sequence. e.g. "I slipped on the lice and broke my arm."
- *Pressure of speech* – Unrelenting, rapid speech without pauses. It may be difficult to interrupt the speaker, and the speaker may continue speaking even when a direct question is asked.

- *Self-reference* – Patient repeatedly and inappropriately refers back to self. e.g. "What's the time?", "It's 7 o'clock. That's my problem."
- *Semantic paraphasia* – Substitution of inappropriate word. e.g. "I slipped on the coat, on the ice I mean, and broke my book."
- *Stilted speech* – Speech characterized by the use of words or phrases that are flowery, excessive, and pompous. e.g. "The attorney comported himself indecorously."
- *Tangentiality* – Wandering from the topic and never returning to it or providing the information requested. e.g. in answer to the question "Where are you from?", a response "My dog is from England. They have good fish and chips there. Fish breathe through gills."
- *Word approximations* – Old words used in a new and unconventional way. e.g. "His boss was a seeover."

Diagnosis

The concept of thought disorder has been criticized as being based on circular or incoherent definitions. For example, thought disorder is inferred from disordered speech, based on the assumption that disordered speech arises because of disordered thought. Incoherence, or word salad, refers to speech that is unconnected and conveys no meaning to the listener.

Furthermore, although thought disorder is typically associated with psychosis, similar phenomena can appear in different disorders, potentially leading to misdiagnosis—for example, in the case of incomplete yet potentially fruitful thought processes.

It has been suggested that individuals with autism spectrum disorders (ASD) display language disturbances like those found in schizophrenia; a 2008 study found that children and adolescents with ASD showed significantly more illogical thinking and loose associations than control subjects. The illogical thinking was related to cognitive functioning and executive control; the loose associations were related to communication symptoms and to parent reports of stress and anxiety.

Delusion

A delusion is a belief that is held with strong conviction despite superior evidence to the contrary. As a pathology, it is distinct from a belief based on false or incomplete information, confabulation, dogma, illusion, or other effects of perception.

Delusions typically occur in the context of neurological or psychiatric disease, although they are not tied to any particular disorder and have been found to occur in the context of many pathological states (both physical and mental). However, they are of particular diagnostic importance in psychotic disorders including schizophrenia, paraphrenia, manic episodes of bipolar disorder, and psychotic depression.

Definition

Although non-specific concepts of madness have been around for several thousand years, the psychiatrist and philosopher Karl Jaspers was the first to define the three main criteria for a belief to be considered delusional in his 1913 book *General Psychopathology*. These criteria are:

- certainty (held with absolute conviction)
- incorrigibility (not changeable by compelling counterargument or proof to the contrary)
- impossibility or falsity of content (implausible, bizarre, or patently untrue)

Furthermore, when a false belief involves a value judgment, it is only considered a delusion if it is so extreme that it cannot be, or never can be proven true. For example: a man claiming that he flew into the sun and flew back home. This would be considered a delusion, unless he were speaking figuratively, or if the belief had a cultural or religious source.

Causes

Explaining the causes of delusions continues to be challenging and several theories have been developed. One is the genetic or biological theory, which states that close relatives of people with delusional disorder are at increased risk of delusional traits. Another theory is the dysfunctional cognitive processing, which states that delusions may arise from distorted ways people have of explaining life to themselves. A third theory is called motivated or defensive delusions. This one states that some of those persons who are predisposed might suffer the onset of delusional disorder in those moments when coping with life and maintaining high self-esteem becomes a significant challenge. In this case, the person views others as the cause of their personal difficulties in order to preserve a positive self-view.

This condition is more common among people who have poor hearing or sight. Also, ongoing stressors have been associated with a higher possibility of developing delusions. Examples of such stressors are immigration, low socioeconomic status, and even possibly the accumulation of smaller daily hassles.

Specific Delusions

The top two factors mainly concerned in the germination of delusions are: 1. Disorder of brain functioning; and 2. background influences of temperament and personality.

Higher levels of dopamine qualify as a symptom of disorders of brain function. That they are needed to sustain certain delusions was examined by a preliminary study on delusional disorder (a psychotic syndrome) instigated to clarify if schizophrenia had a dopamine psychosis. There were positive results - delusions of jealousy and persecution had different levels of dopamine metabolite HVA and homovanillyl alcohol (which may have been genetic). These can be only regarded as tentative results; the study called for future research with a larger population.

It is too simplistic to say that a certain measure of dopamine will bring about a specific delusion. Studies show age and gender to be influential and it is most likely that HVA levels change during the life course of some syndromes.

On the influence personality, it has been said: “Jaspers considered there is a subtle change in personality due to the illness itself; and this creates the condition for the development of the delusional atmosphere in which the delusional intuition arises.”

Cultural factors have “a decisive influence in shaping delusions”. For example, delusions of guilt and punishment are frequent in a Western, Christian country like Austria, but not in Pakistan - where it is more likely persecution. Similarly, in a series of case studies, delusions of guilt and punishment were found in Austrian patients with Parkinson’s being treated with l-dopa - a dopamine agonist.

Types

Delusions are categorized into four different groups:

- Bizarre delusion: Delusions are deemed bizarre if they are clearly implausible and not understandable to same-culture peers and do not derive from ordinary life experiences. An example named by the DSM-5 is a belief that someone replaced all of one’s internal organs with someone else’s without leaving a scar.
- Non-bizarre delusion: A delusion that, though false, is at least possible, e.g., the affected person mistakenly believes that he is under constant police surveillance.
- Mood-congruent delusion: Any delusion with content consistent with either a depressive or manic state, e.g., a depressed person believes that news anchors on television highly disapprove of him, or a person in a manic state might believe she is a powerful deity.
- Mood-neutral delusion: A delusion that does not relate to the sufferer’s emotional state; for example, a belief that an extra limb is growing out of the back of one’s head is neutral to either depression or mania.

Themes

In addition to these categories, delusions often manifest according to a consistent theme. Although delusions can have any theme, certain themes are more common. Some of the more common delusion themes are:

- Delusion of control: False belief that another person, group of people, or external force controls one's general thoughts, feelings, impulses, or behavior.
- Cotard delusion: False belief that one does not exist or has died.
- Delusional jealousy: False belief that a spouse or lover is having an affair, with no proof to back up their claim.
- Delusion of guilt or sin (or delusion of self-accusation): Ungrounded feeling of remorse or guilt of delusional intensity.
- Delusion of mind being read: False belief that other people can know one's thoughts.
- Delusion of thought insertion: Belief that another thinks through the mind of the person.
- Delusion of reference: False belief that insignificant remarks, events, or objects in one's environment have personal meaning or significance.
- Erotomania: False belief that another person is in love with them.
- Grandiose religious delusion: Belief that the affected person is a god or chosen to act as a god.
- Somatic delusion: Delusion whose content pertains to bodily functioning, bodily sensations or physical appearance. Usually the false belief is that the body is somehow diseased, abnormal or changed. A specific example of this delusion is delusional parasitosis: Delusion in which one feels infested with insects, bacteria, mites, spiders, lice, fleas, worms, or other organisms. Affected individuals may also report being repeatedly bitten. In some cases, entomologists are asked to investigate cases of mysterious bites. Sometimes physical manifestations may occur including skin lesions.
- Delusion of poverty: Person strongly believes they are financially incapacitated. Although this type of delusion is less common now, it was particularly widespread in the days preceding state support.

Grandiose delusions or delusions of grandeur are principally a subtype of delusional disorder but could possibly feature as a symptom of schizophrenia and manic episodes of bipolar disorder. Grandiose delusions are characterized by fantastical beliefs that one is famous, omnipotent or otherwise very powerful. The delusions are generally fantastic, often with a supernatural, science-fictional, or religious bent. In colloquial usage, one who overestimates one's own abilities, talents, stature or situation is sometimes said to have "delusions of grandeur". This is generally due to excessive pride, rather than any actual delusions. Grandiose delusions or delusions of grandeur can also be associated with megalomania.

Persecutory Delusions

Persecutory delusions are the most common type of delusions and involve the theme of being followed, harassed, cheated, poisoned or drugged, conspired against, spied on, attacked, or otherwise obstructed in the pursuit of goals. Persecutory delusions are a condition in which the affected person wrongly believes that they are being persecuted. Specifically, they have been defined as containing three central elements: The individual thinks that:

1. harm is occurring, or is going to occur.
2. the persecutor(s) has(have) the intention to cause harm.
3. they are constantly being prejudged or profiled.

According to the DSM-IV-TR, persecutory delusions are the most common form of delusions in schizophrenia, where the person believes they are "being tormented, followed, sabotaged, tricked, spied on, or ridiculed." In the DSM-IV-TR, persecutory delusions are the main feature of the persecutory type of delusional disorder. When the focus is to remedy some injustice by legal action, they are sometimes called "querulous paranoia".

Diagnosis

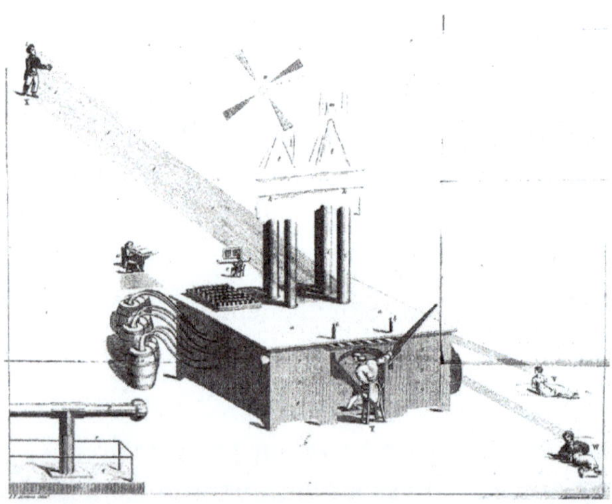

John Haslam illustrated this picture of a machine described by James Tilly Matthews called an "air loom," which Matthews believed was being used to torture him and others for political purposes.

The modern definition and Jaspers' original criteria have been criticised, as counter-examples can be shown for every defining feature.

Studies on psychiatric patients show that delusions vary in intensity and conviction over time, which suggests that certainty and incorrigibility are not necessary components of a delusional belief.

Delusions do not necessarily have to be false or 'incorrect inferences about external reality'. Some religious or spiritual beliefs by their nature may not be falsifiable, and hence cannot be described as false or incorrect, no matter whether the person holding these beliefs was diagnosed as delusional or not.

In other situations the delusion may turn out to be true belief. For example, in delusional jealousy, where a person believes that their partner is being unfaithful (and may even follow them into the bathroom believing them to be seeing their lover even during the briefest of partings), it may actually be true that the partner is having sexual relations with another person. In this case, the delusion does not cease to be a delusion because the content later turns out to be verified as true or the partner actually chose to engage in the behavior of which they were being accused.

In other cases, the delusion may be assumed to be false by a doctor or psychiatrist assessing the belief, because it *seems* to be unlikely, bizarre or held with excessive conviction. Psychiatrists rarely have the time or resources to check the validity of a person's claims leading to some true beliefs to be erroneously classified as delusional. This is known as the Martha Mitchell effect, after the wife of the attorney general who alleged that illegal activity was taking place in the White House. At the time, her claims were thought to be signs of mental illness, and only after the Watergate scandal broke was she proved right (and hence sane).

Similar factors have led to criticisms of Jaspers' definition of true delusions as being ultimately 'un-understandable'. Critics (such as R. D. Laing) have argued that this leads to the diagnosis of delusions being based on the subjective understanding of a particular psychiatrist, who may not have access to all the information that might make a belief otherwise interpretable. R. D. Laing's hypothesis has been applied to some forms of projective therapy to "fix" a delusional system so that it cannot be altered by the patient. Psychiatric researchers at Yale University, Ohio State University and the Community Mental Health Center of Middle Georgia have used novels and motion picture films as the focus. Texts, plots and cinematography are discussed and the delusions approached tangentially. This use of fiction to decrease the malleability of a delusion was employed in a joint project by science-fiction author Philip Jose Farmer and Yale psychiatrist A. James Giannini. They wrote the novel *Red Orc's Rage*, which, recursively, deals with delusional adolescents who are treated with a form of projective therapy. In this novel's fictional setting other novels written by Farmer are discussed and the characters are symbolically integrated into the delusions of fictional patients. This particular novel was then applied to real-life clinical settings.

Another difficulty with the diagnosis of delusions is that almost all of these features can be found in "normal" beliefs. Many religious beliefs hold exactly the same features, yet are not universally considered delusional. These factors have led the psychiatrist Anthony David to note that "there is no acceptable (rather than accepted) definition of a delusion." In practice, psychiatrists tend to diagnose a belief as delusional if it is either patently bizarre, causing significant distress, or excessively pre-occupying the patient, especially if the person is subsequently unswayed in belief by counter-evidence or reasonable arguments.

It is important to distinguish true delusions from other symptoms such as anxiety, fear, or paranoia. To diagnose delusions a mental state examination may be used. This test includes appearance, mood, affect, behavior, rate and continuity of speech, evidence of hallucinations or abnormal beliefs, thought content, orientation to time, place and person, attention and concentration, insight and judgment, as well as short-term memory.

Johnson-Laird suggests that delusions may be viewed as the natural consequence of failure to distinguish conceptual relevance. That is, the person takes irrelevant information and puts it in the form of disconnected experiences, then it is taken to be relevant in a manner that suggests false causal connections. Furthermore, the person takes the relevant information, in the form of counterexamples, and ignores it.

Treatment

Psychotherapies that may be helpful in delusional disorder include individual psychotherapy, cognitive-behavioral therapy (CBT), and family therapy.

Diagnosis of Schizophrenia

The diagnosis of schizophrenia is based on criteria in either the American Psychiatric Association's *Diagnostic and Statistical Manual of Mental Disorders,* version DSM-IV-TR, or the World Health Organization's International Statistical Classification of Diseases and Related Health Problems, the ICD-10. These criteria use the self-reported experiences of the person and reported abnormalities in behavior, followed by a clinical assessment by a mental health professional. Symptoms associated with schizophrenia occur along a continuum in the population and must reach a certain severity before a diagnosis is made.

Criteria

The ICD-10 criteria are typically used in most of the world, while the DSM-IV-TR and DSM-5 criteria are used in USA, ICD is prevailing in research studies. The ICD-10 criteria put more emphasis on Schneiderian first-rank symptoms. In practice, agreement between the two systems is high.

According to the revised fourth edition of the *Diagnostic and Statistical Manual of Mental Disorders* (DSM-IV-TR), to be diagnosed with schizophrenia, three diagnostic criteria must be met:

1. Characteristic symptoms: Two or more of the following, each present for much of the time during a one-month period (or less, if symptoms remitted with treatment).
   - Delusions
   - Hallucinations
   - Disorganized speech, which is a manifestation of formal thought disorder
   - Grossly disorganized behavior (e.g. dressing inappropriately, crying frequently) or catatonic behavior
   - Negative symptoms: Blunted affect (lack or decline in emotional response), alogia (lack or decline in speech), or avolition (lack or decline in motivation)

   If the delusions are judged to be bizarre, or hallucinations consist of hearing one voice participating in a running commentary of the patient's actions or of hearing two or more voices conversing with each other, only that symptom is required above. The speech disorganization criterion is only met if it is severe enough to substantially impair communication.

2. Social or occupational dysfunction: For a significant portion of the time since the onset of the disturbance, one or more major areas of functioning such as work, interpersonal relations, or self-care, are markedly below the level achieved prior to the onset.

3. Significant duration: Continuous signs of the disturbance persist for at least six months. This six-month period must include at least one month of symptoms (or less, if symptoms remitted with treatment).

If signs of disturbance are present for more than a month but less than six months, the diagnosis of schizophreniform disorder is applied. Psychotic symptoms lasting less than a month may be diagnosed as brief psychotic disorder, and various conditions may be classed as psychotic disorder not otherwise specified. Schizophrenia cannot be diagnosed if symptoms of mood disorder are substantially present (although schizoaffective disorder could be diagnosed), or if symptoms of pervasive developmental disorder are present unless prominent delusions or hallucinations are also present, or if the symptoms are the direct physiological result of a general medical condition or a substance, such as abuse of a drug or medication.

Subtypes

The DSM-IV-TR contains five sub-classifications of schizophrenia, although the developers of DSM-5 are recommending they be dropped from the new classification:

- Paranoid type: Where delusions and hallucinations are present but thought disorder, disorganized behavior, and affective flattening are absent. (DSM code 295.3/ICD code F20.0)

- Disorganized type: Named *hebephrenic schizophrenia* in the ICD. Where thought disorder and flat affect are present together. (DSM code 295.1/ICD code F20.1)
- Catatonic type: The subject may be almost immobile or exhibit agitated, purposeless movement. Symptoms can include catatonic stupor and waxy flexibility. (DSM code 295.2/ICD code F20.2)
- Undifferentiated type: Psychotic symptoms are present but the criteria for paranoid, disorganized, or catatonic types have not been met. (DSM code 295.9/ ICD code F20.3)
- Residual type: Where positive symptoms are present at a low intensity only. (DSM code 295.6/ICD code F20.5)

The ICD-10 defines two additional subtypes:

- Post-schizophrenic depression: A depressive episode arising in the aftermath of a schizophrenic illness where some low-level schizophrenic symptoms may still be present. (ICD code F20.4)
- Simple schizophrenia: Insidious and progressive development of prominent negative symptoms with no history of psychotic episodes. (ICD code F20.6)

Differential

Psychotic symptoms may be present in several other mental disorders, including bipolar disorder, borderline personality disorder, drug intoxication and drug-induced psychosis. Delusions ("non-bizarre") are also present in delusional disorder, and social withdrawal in social anxiety disorder, avoidant personality disorder and schizotypal personality disorder. Schizophrenia is complicated with obsessive-compulsive disorder (OCD) considerably more often than could be explained by pure chance, although it can be difficult to distinguish obsessions that occur in OCD from the delusions of schizophrenia.

A more general medical and neurological examination may be needed to rule out medical illnesses which may rarely produce psychotic schizophrenia-like symptoms, such as metabolic disturbance, systemic infection, syphilis, HIV infection, epilepsy, and brain lesions. It may be necessary to rule out a delirium, which can be distinguished by visual hallucinations, acute onset and fluctuating level of consciousness, and indicates an underlying medical illness. Investigations are not generally repeated for relapse unless there is a specific *medical* indication or possible adverse effects from antipsychotic medication.

"Schizophrenia" does *not* mean dissociative identity disorder—formerly and still widely known as "multiple personalities"—despite the etymology of the word.

Early, Late, and Very Late Onset

Early-onset schizophrenia refers to individuals who had their first episode of symptoms at age 20-30. Late-onset refers to those whose first episode of symptoms began after the age of 40. Very-late-onset refers to those with their first episode of symptoms at age 60 and older. It is estimated that 15% of the population with schizophrenia are late-onset and 5% are very-late onset.

Many of the symptoms of late-onset schizophrenia are similar to the early-onset. However, individuals with late-onsets are more likely to report:

- Visual, tactile, and olfactory hallucinations
- Persecutory delusion
- Partition delusions
- Third-person, running commentary
- Accusatory or abusive auditory hallucinations

Late-onsets are less likely to have:

- Formal thought disorder
- Affective flattening or blunting
- Paranoia

Very late-onset are likely to have:

- Less formal thought disorder or cognitive impairment
- Fewer negative symptoms

Controversies

There is an argument that the underlying issues would be better addressed as a spectrum of conditions or as individual dimensions along which everyone varies rather than by a diagnostic category based on an arbitrary cut-off between normal and ill. This approach appears consistent with research on schizotypy, and with a relatively high prevalence of psychotic experiences, mostly non-distressing delusional beliefs, among the general public. In concordance with this observation, psychologist Edgar Jones, and psychiatrists Tony David and Nassir Ghaemi, surveying the existing literature on delusions, pointed out that the consistency and completeness of the definition of delusion have been found wanting by many; delusions are neither necessarily fixed nor false, and need not involve the presence of incontrovertible evidence.

Nancy Andreasen has criticized the current DSM-IV and ICD-10 criteria for sacrificing diagnostic validity for the sake of artificially improving reliability. She argues that over-emphasis on psychosis in the diagnostic criteria, while improving diagnostic reliability, ignores more fundamental cognitive impairments that are harder to assess due to large variations in presentation. This view is supported by other psychiatrists. In the same vein, Ming Tsuang and colleagues argue that psychotic symptoms may be a common end-state in a variety of disorders, including schizophrenia, rather than a reflection of the specific etiology of schizophrenia, and warn that there is little basis for regarding DSM's operational definition as the "true" construct of schizophrenia. Neuropsychologist Michael Foster Green went further in suggesting the presence of specific neurocognitive deficits may be used to construct phenotypes that are alternatives to those that are purely symptom-based. These deficits take the form of a reduction or impairment in basic psychological functions such as memory, attention, executive function and problem solving.

The exclusion of affective components from the criteria for schizophrenia, despite their ubiquity in clinical settings, has also caused contention. This exclusion in the DSM has resulted in a "rather convoluted" separate disorder—schizoaffective disorder. Citing poor interrater reliability, some psychiatrists have totally contested the concept of schizoaffective disorder as a separate entity. The categorical distinction between mood disorders and schizophrenia, known as the Kraepelinian dichotomy, has also been challenged by data from genetic epidemiology.

Causes of Schizophrenia

The causes of schizophrenia have been the subject of much debate, with various factors proposed and discounted or modified. The language of schizophrenia research under the medical model is scientific. Such studies suggest that genetics, prenatal development, early environment, neurobiology and psychological and social processes are important contributory factors. Current psychiatric research into the development of the disorder is often based on a neurodevelopmental model. However, schizophrenia is diagnosed on the basis of symptom profiles. Neural correlates do not provide sufficiently useful criteria. "Current research into schizophrenia has remained highly fragmented, much like the clinical presentation of the disease itself". The one thing that researchers can agree on is that schizophrenia is a complicated and variable condition. It is best thought of as a syndrome, a cluster of symptoms that may or may not have related causes, rather than a single disease.

It is possible for schizophrenia to develop at any age, but it mostly happens to people within the ages of 16–30 (generally males 16–25 and females 25–30) - about 75 percent of people living with the illness develop it at this age. There is a likelihood of children developing schizophrenia, though it is quite rare before the age of 12. Also, new cases are uncommon after age 40. In addition, about 1 percent of the world's population will develop schizophrenia over their lifetime, therefore out of all the people born, one in 100 will develop schizophrenia by age 55. There is on average a somewhat earlier onset for men than women, with the possible influence of the female hormone estrogen being one hypothesis and sociocultural influences another.

Genetics

Heritability

Evidence suggests that genetic vulnerability with environmental factors can act in combination resulting in the development of schizophrenia. Although schizophrenia is very strongly heritable, there is also some evidence that all cases are not caused by heredity. Many people who appear to carry "schizophrenia genes" may not become schizophrenic. Recent research suggests that genetic vulnerability to schizophrenia is multifactorial, caused by interactions of several genes.

Individual twin studies and meta-analyses of twin studies have estimated the heritability of risk for schizophrenia to be approximately 80% (this refers to the proportion of variation between individuals in a population that is influenced by genetic factors, not the degree of genetic determination of individual risk), but the heritability estimate varies from 41 to 87%. Concordance rates between monozygotic twins vary in different studies, approximately 50%; whereas dizygotic twins was 17%. Some twin studies have found rates as low as 11.0%–13.8% among monozygotic twins, and 1.8%–4.1% among dizygotic twins, however.

Family studies indicate that the closer a person's genetic relatedness to a person with schizophrenia, the greater the likelihood of developing the disorder. The paternal age is a factor in schizophrenia because of the increased likelihood of mutations in the chromosomes of cells that produce sperms. In contrast, women's oocytes divide twenty-three times before the time of birth and only once after that. The chance of a copying error in DNA replication during cell division increases with the number of cell divisions, and an increase in copying errors may cause an accumulation of mutations that are responsible for an increased incidence of schizophrenia. The average concordance rates are higher for identical twins than for fraternal twins and evidence also suggests that the prenatal and perinatal environments may also affect concordance rates in identical twins.

Genetic Candidates

Although twin studies and family studies have indicated a large degree of heritability for schizophrenia, the exact genetic causes remain unclear. Recently however, quite some large-scale studies have now begun to unravel the genetic underpinnings for the disease. Important segregation should be made between lower risk, common variants (identified by candidate studies or genome-wide association studies(GWAS)) and high risk, rare variants (which could be caused by de novo mutations) and copy-number variations (CNVs).

Candidate Gene Studies

An older 2003 review of linkage studies also listed seven genes as likely to increase risk for a later diagnosis of the disorder. Two recent reviews suggested that the evidence was strongest for two genes known as dysbindin (*DTNBP1*) and neuregulin (NRG1), and that a number of other genes (such as *COMT*, *RGS4*, *PPP3CC*, *ZDHHC8*, *DISC1*, and *AKT1*) showed some early promising results. Knockout studies in *Drosophila* show that reduced expression of dysbindin reduced glutamatergic synaptic transmission, resulting in impaired memory. Variations near the gene *FXYD6* have also been associated with schizophrenia in the UK but not in Japan. In 2008, rs7341475 SNP of the reelin gene was associated with an increased risk of schizophrenia in women, but not in men. This female-specific association was replicated in several populations. Still another review found evidence that the protein phosphatase 2B (calcineurin) might be involved in susceptibility to schizophrenia.

The largest most comprehensive genetic study of its kind, involving tests of several hundred single nucleotide polymorphisms (SNPs) in nearly 1,900 individuals with schizophrenia or schizoaffective disorder and 2,000 comparison subjects, reported in 2008 that there was no evidence of any significant association between the disorders and any of 14 previously identified candidate genes (*RGS4*, *DISC1*, *DTNBP1*, *STX7*, *TAAR6*, *PPP3CC*, *NRG1*, *DRD2*, *HTR2A*, *DAOA*, *AKT1*, *CHRNA7*, *COMT*, and *ARVCF*). The statistical distributions suggested nothing more than chance variation. The authors concluded that the findings make it unlikely that common SNPs in these genes account for a substantial proportion of the genetic risk for schizophrenia, although small effects could not be ruled out.

The perhaps largest analysis of genetic associations in schizophrenia is with the *SzGene* database at the *Schizophrenia Research Forum*. One 2008 meta-analysis examined genetic variants in 16 genes and found nominally significant effects.

A 2009 study was able to create mice matching schizophrenic symptoms by the deletion of only one gene set, those of the neuregulin post-synaptic receptor. The result showed that although the mice mostly developed normally, on further brain development, glutamate receptors broke down. This theory supports the glutamate hypothesis of schizophrenia. Another study in 2009 by Simon Fraser University researchers identifies a link between autism and schizophrenia: "The SFU group found that variations in four sets of genes are related to both autism and schizophrenia. People normally have two copies of each gene, but in autistics some genome locations have only single copies and in schizophrenics extra copies are present at the same locations."

Genome-wide Association Studies

To increase sample size for a better powered detection of common variants with small effects, GWAS data is continuing to be clustered in large international consortia. The

Psychiatric Genetics Consortium (PGC) attempts to aggregate GWAS data on schizophrenia to detect associations of common variants with small effect on disease risk.

In 2011, this collaboration identified by meta-analyse of genome-wide association studies that 129 over 136 single-nucleotide polymorphism (SNP) significantly associated with schizophrenia were located in major histocompatibility complex region of the genome.

In 2013 this dataset was expanded to identify in total 13 candidate loci for the disease, now also implicating calcium signalling as an important factor in the disease.

In 2014 this collaboration expanded to an even larger meta-analysis, the largest to date, on GWAS data (36,989 cases and 113,075 controls) in *Nature*, indicating 108 schizophrenia-associated genetic loci, of which 83 have not been previously described. Together, these candidate genes pointed to an importance of neurotransmission and immunology as important factors in the disease.

Distinct symptomatic subtypes of schizophrenia groups showed to have a different pattern of SNP variations, reflecting the heterogeneous nature of the disease.

A 2016 study implicated the C4 gene in schizophrenia risk. C4 was found to play a role in synapse pruning, and increased C4 expression leads to reduced dendritic spines and a higher schizophrenia risk.

Copy-number Variations

Other research has suggested that a greater than average number of structural variations such as rare deletions or duplications of tiny DNA sequences within genes (known as copy number variants) are linked to increased risk for schizophrenia, especially in "sporadic" cases not linked to family history of schizophrenia, and that the genetic factors and developmental pathways can thus be different in different individuals. A genome wide survey of 3,391 individuals with schizophrenia found CNVs in less than 1% of cases. Within them, deletions in regions related to psychosis were observed, as well as deletions on chromosome 15q13.3 and 1q21.1.

CNVs occur due to non-allelic homologous recombination mediated by low copy repeats (sequentially similar regions). This results in deletions and duplications of dosage sensitive genes. It has been speculated that CNVs underlie a significant proportion of normal human variation, including differences in cognitive, behavioral, and psychological features, and that CNVs in at least three loci can result in increased risk for schizophrenia in a few individuals. Epigenetics may also play a role in schizophrenia, with the expression of Protocadherin 11 X/Protocadherin Y playing a possible role in schizophrenia.

A 2008 investigation of 2,977 schizophrenia patients and 33,746 controls from seven European populations examined CNVs in neurexins, and found that exon-affecting deletions in the NRXN1 gene conferred risk of schizophrenia.

An updated meta-analysis on CNVs for schizophrenia published in 2015 expanded the number of CNVs indicated in the disease, which was also the first genetic evidence for the involvement of GABAergic neurotransmission. This study further supported genetic involvement for excitatory neurotransmission.

Overlap with Other Disorders

Several studies have suggested that genetic overlap exists between schizophrenia and other psychiatric disorders. In February 28, 2013 The Lancet published an article about the possible genetic correlation between autism spectrum disorder, attention deficit-hyperactivity disorder, bipolar disorder, major depressive disorder, and schizophrenia. They analyzed genome-wide single-nucleotide polymorphism (SNP) data for the five disorders in 33 332 cases and 27 888 controls of European ancestry. This group found four gene areas that all overlapped with the five disorders, two of which regulate calcium balance in the brain.

Evolutionary Psychology

Schizophrenia has been considered an evolutionary puzzle due to the combination of high heritability, relatively high prevalence, and reduced reproductive success. One explanation could be increased reproductive success by close relatives without symptoms but this does not seem to be the case. Still, it has been argued that it is possible that a low amount of schizotypy increasing genes may increase reproductive success by increasing such traits such as creativity, verbal ability, and emotional sensitivity.

Another evolutionary explanation is the "imprinted brain theory" which argues that psychosis and autism are contrasting disorders on a number of different variables. This is argued to be caused by an unbalanced genomic imprinting favoring paternal genes in the case of autism and maternal genes in the case of psychosis.

Before Birth

It is well established that obstetric complications or events are associated with an increased chance of the child later developing schizophrenia, although overall they constitute a non-specific risk factor with a relatively small effect. Obstetric complications occur in approximately 25 to 30% of the general population and the vast majority do not develop schizophrenia, and likewise the majority of individuals with schizophrenia have not had a detectable obstetric event. Nevertheless, the increased average risk is well-replicated, and such events may moderate the effects of genetic or other environmental risk factors. The specific complications or events most linked to schizophrenia, and the mechanisms of their effects, are still under examination.

One epidemiological finding is that people diagnosed with schizophrenia are more likely to have been born in winter or spring (at least in the northern hemisphere). However, the effect is not large. Explanations have included a greater prevalence of viral infections at that time, or a greater likelihood of vitamin D deficiency. A similar effect (increased likelihood of being born in winter and spring) has also been found with other, healthy populations, such as chess players.

Women who were pregnant during the Dutch famine of 1944, where many people were close to starvation (experiencing malnutrition) had a higher chance of having a child who would later develop schizophrenia. Studies of Finnish mothers who were pregnant when they found out that their husbands had been killed during the Winter War of 1939–1940 have shown that their children were significantly more likely to develop schizophrenia when compared with mothers who found out about their husbands' death after pregnancy, suggesting that maternal stress may have an effect.

Fetal Growth

Lower than average birth weight has been one of the most consistent findings, indicating slowed fetal growth possibly mediated by genetic effects. In the first and only prospective study of the low birthweight, schizophrenia, and enlargement of brain ventricles suggestive of cerebral atrophy, Leigh Silverton and colleagues found that low birthweight (measured prospectively with regard to psychopathology) was associated with enlarged ventricles on CT-Scans in a sample at risk for schizophrenia over 30 years later. These signs suggestive of cerebral atrophy were associated with schizophrenia symptoms. In a follow up study, Silverton et al. noted an interaction between genetic risk for schizophrenia and low birthweight. The risk of enlarged ventricles on brain scan (associated with schizophrenia symptoms and biologically suggestive of Emil Kraepelin's dementia praecox type of schizophrenia) was greatly increased if the subjects had both a higher genetic load for schizophrenia and lower birthweight. The investigators suggested that in utero insults may specifically stress those with a schizophrenia diathesis suggesting to the authors a diathesis stress etiological model for a certain type of schizophrenia (that Kraepelin identified) with early abnormalities suggesting brain atrophy.

Some investigators have noted, however, that any factor adversely affecting the fetus will affect growth rate, however, so believe that this association has may not be particularly informative regarding causation. In addition, the majority of birth cohort studies have failed to find a link between schizophrenia and low birth weight or other signs of growth retardation. It should be noted, however, that the majority of studies do not measure the interaction of genetic risk and birthweight as was done in the Silverton et al. studies.

Hypoxia

It has been hypothesized since the 1970s that brain hypoxia (low oxygen levels) before, at or immediately after birth may be a risk factor for the development of schizophrenia.

Hypoxia is now being demonstrated as relevant to schizophrenia in animal models, molecular biology and epidemiology studies. One study in Molecular Psychiatry was able to differentiate 90% of schizophrenics from controls based on hypoxia and metabolism. Hypoxia has been recently described as one of the most important of the external factors that influence susceptibility, although studies have been mainly epidemiological. Such studies place a high degree of importance on hypoxic influence, but because of familial pattern of the illness in some families, propose a genetic factor also; stopping short of concluding hypoxia to be the sole cause. Fetal hypoxia, in the presence of certain unidentified genes, has been correlated with reduced volume of the hippocampus, which is in turn correlated with schizophrenia.

Although most studies have interpreted hypoxia as causing some form of neuronal dysfunction or even subtle damage, it has been suggested that the physiological hypoxia that prevails in normal embryonic and fetal development, or pathological hypoxia or ischemia, may exert an effect by regulating or dysregulating genes involved in neurodevelopment. A literature review judged that over 50% of the candidate genes for susceptibility to schizophrenia met criteria for "ischemia–hypoxia regulation or vascular expression" even though only 3.5% of all genes were estimated to be involved in hypoxia/ischemia or the vasculature.

A longitudinal study found that obstetric complications involving hypoxia were one factor associated with neurodevelopmental impairments in childhood and with the later development of schizophreniform disorders. Fetal hypoxia has been found to predict unusual movements at age 4 (but not age 7) among children who go on to develop schizophrenia, suggesting that its effects are specific to the stage of neurodevelopment. A Japanese case study of monozygotic twins discordant for schizophrenia (one has the diagnosis while the other does not) draws attention to their different weights at birth and concludes hypoxia may be the differentiating factor.

The unusual functional laterality in speech production (e.g. right hemisphere auditory processing) found in some individuals with schizophrenia could be due to aberrant neural networks established as a compensation for left temporal lobe damage induced by pre- or perinatal hypoxia. Prenatal and perinatal hypoxia appears to be important as one factor in the neurodevelopmental model, with the important implication that some forms of schizophrenia may thus be preventable.

Research on rodents seeking to understand the possible role of prenatal hypoxia in disorders such as schizophrenia has indicated that it can lead to a range of sensorimotor and learning/memory abnormalities. Impairments in motor function and coordination, evident on challenging tasks when the hypoxia was severe enough to cause brain damage, were long-lasting and described as a "hallmark of prenatal hypoxia".

Several animal studies have indicated that fetal hypoxia can affect many of the same neural substrates implicated in schizophrenia, depending on the severity and duration of the hypoxic event as well as the period of gestation, and in humans moderate or severe (but not mild) fetal hypoxia has been linked to a series of motor, language and cognitive deficits in children, regardless of genetic liability to schizophrenia. One paper restated that cerebellum neurological disorders were frequently found in schizophrenics and speculated hypoxia may cause the subsequent cognitive dysmetria.

Whereas most studies find only a modest effect of hypoxia in schizophrenia, a longitudinal study using a combination of indicators to detect possible fetal hypoxia, such as early equivalents of Neurological Soft Signs or obstetric complications, reported that the risk of schizophrenia and other nonaffective psychoses was "strikingly elevated" (5.75% versus 0.39%). Although objective estimates of hypoxia did not account for all schizophrenic cases; the study revealed increasing odds of schizophrenia according to graded increase in severity of hypoxia.

Other Factors

There is an emerging literature on a wide range of prenatal risk factors, such as prenatal stress, intrauterine (in the womb) malnutrition, and prenatal infection. Increased paternal age has been linked to schizophrenia, possibly due to "chromosomal aberrations and mutations of the aging germline." Maternal-fetal rhesus or genotype incompatibility has also been linked, via increasing the risk of an adverse prenatal environment. Also, in mothers with schizophrenia, an increased risk has been identified via a complex interaction between maternal genotype, maternal behavior, prenatal environment and possibly medication and socioeconomic factors. References for many of these environmental risk factors have been collected in an online database.

There may be an association between celiac disease (gluten intolerance) and schizophrenia in a small proportion of patients, though large randomized controlled trials and epidemiological studies will be needed before such an association can be confirmed. Withdrawal of gluten from the diet is an inexpensive measure which may improve the symptoms in a small (≤3%) number of schizophrenic patients.

In addition, there is some evidence that exposure to toxins such as lead can also increase the risk of later development of schizophrenia spectrum disorders.

A meta-analysis found that high neuroticism increases the risk of psychosis and schizophrenia.

Infections and Immune System

Numerous viral infections, in utero or in childhood, have been associated with an increased risk of later developing schizophrenia. Schizophrenia is somewhat more common in those born in winter to early spring, when infections are more common.

Influenza has long been studied as a possible factor. A 1988 study found that individuals who were exposed to the Asian flu as second trimester fetuses were at increased risk of eventually developing schizophrenia. This result was corroborated by a later British study of the same pandemic, but not by a 1994 study of the pandemic in Croatia. A Japanese study also found no support for a link between schizophrenia and birth after an influenza epidemic.

Polio, measles, varicella-zoster, rubella, herpes simplex virus type 2, maternal genital infections, Borna disease virus, and more recently *Toxoplasma gondii* have been correlated with the later development of schizophrenia. Psychiatrists E. Fuller Torrey and R.H. Yolken have hypothesized that the latter, a common parasite in humans, contributes to some, if not many, cases of schizophrenia.

In a meta-analysis of several studies, they found moderately higher levels of *Toxoplasma* antibodies in those with schizophrenia and possibly higher rates of prenatal or early postnatal exposure to *Toxoplasma gondii*, but not acute infection. However, in another study of postmortem brain tissue, the authors have reported equivocal or negative results, including no evidence of herpes virus or *T. gondii* involvement in schizophrenia.

There is some evidence for the role of autoimmunity in the development of some cases of schizophrenia. A statistical correlation has been reported with various autoimmune diseases and direct studies have linked dysfunctional immune status to some of the clinical features of schizophrenia.

This is known as the pathogenic theory of schizophrenia or germ theory of schizophrenia. It is a pathogenic theory of disease in which it is thought that a proximal cause of certain cases of schizophrenia is the interaction of the developing fetus with pathogens such as viruses, or with antibodies from the mother created in response to these pathogens (in particular, Interleukin 8). Substantial research suggests that exposure to certain illnesses (e.g., influenza) in the mother of the neonate (especially at the end of the second trimester) causes defects in neural development which may emerge as a predisposition to schizophrenia around the time of puberty, as the brain grows and develops.

Recent findings support the hypothesis that schizophrenia is associated with alterations of the tryptophane-kynurenine metabolic pathway due to activation of specific sections of the immune system.

The relevance of some auto-antibodies that act against the NMDAR and VGKC is being studied. Current estimates suggest that between 1.5 - 6.5% of patients have these antibodies in their blood. Preliminary results have shown that these patients can be treated with immunotherapy such as IVIG or Plasma exchange and steroids, on top of anti-psychotic medication, which can lead to a reduction in symptoms.

Childhood Antecedents

In general, the antecedents of schizophrenia are subtle and those who will go on to develop schizophrenia do not form a readily identifiable subgroup - which would lead to identification of a specific cause. Average group differences from the norm may be in the direction of superior as well as inferior performance. Overall, birth cohort studies have indicated subtle nonspecific behavioral features, some evidence for psychotic-like experiences (particularly hallucinations), and various cognitive antecedents. There have been some inconsistencies in the particular domains of functioning identified and whether they continue through childhood and whether they are specific to schizophrenia.

A prospective study found average differences across a range of developmental domains, including reaching milestones of motor development at a later age, having more speech problems, lower educational test results, solitary play preferences at ages four and six, and being more socially anxious at age 13. Lower ratings of the mother's skills and understanding of the child at age 4 were also related.

Some of the early developmental differences were identified in the first year of life in a study in Finland, although generally related to psychotic disorders rather than schizophrenia in particular. The early subtle motor signs persisted to some extent, showing a small link to later school performance in adolescence. An earlier Finnish study found that childhood performance of 400 individuals diagnosed with schizophrenia was significantly worse than controls on subjects involving motor co-ordination (sports and handcrafts) between ages 7 and 9, but there were no differences on academic subjects (contrary to some other IQ findings). (Patients in this age group with these symptoms were significantly less likely to progress to high school, despite academic ability.)

Symptoms of schizophrenia often appear soon after puberty, when the brain is undergoing significant maturational changes. Some investigators believe that the disease process of schizophrenia begins prenatally, lies dormant until puberty, and then causes a period of neural degeneration that causes the symptoms to emerge. However, reanalysis of the data from the later Finnish study, on older children (14 to 16) in a changed school system, using narrower diagnostic criteria and with less cases but more controls, did not support a significant difference on sports and handicraft performance. However, another study found that unusual motor coordination scores at 7 years of age were associated in adulthood with both those with schizophrenia and their unaffected siblings, while unusual movements at ages 4 and 7 predicted adult schizophrenia but not unaffected sibling status.

A birth cohort study in New Zealand found that children who went on to develop schizophreniform disorder had, as well as emotional problems and interpersonal difficulties linked to all adult psychiatric outcomes measured, significant impairments in neuromotor, receptive language, and cognitive development. A retrospective study found that adults with schizophrenia had performed better than average in artistic subjects at ages 12 and 15, and in linguistic and religious subjects at age 12, but worse than average in gymnastics at age 15.

Some small studies on offspring of individuals with schizophrenia have identified various neurobehavioral deficits, a poorer family environment and disruptive school behaviour, poor peer engagement, immaturity or unpopularity or poorer social competence and increasing schizophrenic symptomology emerging during adolescence.

A minority "deficit syndrome" subtype of schizophrenia is proposed to be more marked by early poor adjustment and behavioral problems, as compared to non-deficit subtypes.

There is evidence that childhood experiences of abuse or trauma are risk factors for a diagnosis of schizophrenia later in life. Some researchers reported that hallucinations and other symptoms considered characteristic of schizophrenia and psychosis were at least as strongly related to neglect and childhood abuse as many other mental health problems. The researchers concluded that there is a need for staff training in asking patients about abuse, and a need to offer appropriate psychosocial treatments to those who have been neglected and abused as children.

Substance Use

The relationship between schizophrenia and drug use is complex, meaning that a clear causal connection between drug use and schizophrenia has been difficult to tease apart. Some substances can induce psychosis. The use of various drugs makes a diagnosis of schizophrenia more complicated. A person cannot be diagnosed without symptoms persisting after drug use have ended. There is strong evidence that using certain drugs can trigger either the onset or relapse of schizophrenia in some people. It may also be the case, however, that people with schizophrenia use drugs to overcome negative feelings associated with both the commonly prescribed antipsychotic medication and the condition itself, where negative emotion, paranoia and anhedonia are all considered to be core features.

The rate of substance use is known to be particularly high in this group. In a recent study, 60% of people with schizophrenia were found to use substances and 37% would be diagnosable with a substance use disorder.

Cannabis

There is some evidence that cannabis use can contribute to schizophrenia. Some studies suggest that cannabis is neither a sufficient nor necessary factor in developing schizophrenia, but that cannabis may significantly increase the risk of developing schizophrenia and may be, among other things, a significant causal factor. Nevertheless, some previous research in this area has been criticised as it has often not been clear whether cannabis use is a cause or effect of schizophrenia. To address this issue, a recent review of prospective cohort studies has suggested that cannabis statistically doubles the risk of developing schizophrenia on the individual level, and may, if a causal relationship is assumed, be responsible for up to 8% of cases in the population.

Cannabis misuse by young people is suspected of causing schizophrenia in later life by interfering with and distorting neurodevelopment particularly of the prefrontal cortex region of the brain. An older longitudinal study, published in 1987, suggested a sixfold increase of schizophrenia risks for high consumers of cannabis (use on more than fifty occasions) in Sweden.

Cannabis use is also suspected to contribute to the hyperdopaminergic state that is characteristic of schizophrenia. Compounds found in cannabis, such as THC, have been shown to increase the activity of dopamine pathways in the brain, suggesting that cannabis may exacerbate symptoms of psychosis in schizophrenics.

Despite increases in cannabis consumption in the 1960s and 1970s in western society, rates of psychotic disorders such as schizophrenia remained relatively stable over time.

Amphetamines and Other Stimulants

As amphetamines trigger the release of dopamine and excessive dopamine function is believed to be responsible for many symptoms of schizophrenia (known as the dopamine hypothesis of schizophrenia), amphetamines may worsen schizophrenia symptoms. Methamphetamine, a potent neurotoxic amphetamine derivative, induces psychosis in a substantial minority of regular users which resembles paranoid schizophrenia. For most people, this psychosis fades away within a month of abstinence but for a minority the psychosis can become chronic. Individuals who develop a long lasting psychosis, despite abstinence from methamphetamine, more commonly have a family history of schizophrenia.

Concerns have been raised that long-term therapy with stimulants for ADHD might cause paranoia, schizophrenia and behavioral sensitization. Family history of mental illness does not predict the incidence of stimulant toxicosis in ADHD children. High rates of childhood stimulant use have been noted in patients with a diagnosis of schizophrenia and bipolar disorder independent of ADHD. Individuals with a diagnosis of bipolar or schizophrenia who were prescribed stimulants during childhood typically have a significantly earlier onset of the psychotic disorder and suffer a more severe clinical course of psychotic disorder. It has been suggested that this small subgroup of children who develop schizophrenia due to stimulant use during childhood have a genetic vulnerability to developing psychosis. In addition, amphetamines are known to cause a stimulant psychosis in otherwise healthy individuals that superficially resembles schizophrenia, and may be misdiagnosed as such by some healthcare professionals.

Hallucinogens

Drugs such as ketamine, PCP, and LSD have been used to mimic schizophrenia for research purposes. Using LSD and other psychedelics as a model has now fallen out of favor with the scientific research community, as the differences between the drug induced states and the typical presentation of schizophrenia have become clear. The dissociatives ketamine and PCP, however, are still considered to produce states that are remarkably similar, and are considered to be even better models than stimulants since they produce both positive and negative symptoms.

Alcohol

Approximately three percent of people who are alcohol dependent experience psychosis during acute intoxication or withdrawal. The mechanism of alcohol-related psychosis is due to distortions to neuronal membranes, gene expression, as well as thiamin deficiency. There is evidence that alcohol abuse via a kindling mechanism can occasionally cause the development of a chronic substance induced psychotic disorder, i.e. schizophrenia.

Tobacco Use

People with schizophrenia tend to smoke significantly more tobacco than the general population. The rates are exceptionally high amongst institutionalized patients and homeless people. In a UK census from 1993, 74% of people with schizophrenia living in institutions were found to be smokers. A 1999 study that covered all people with schizophrenia in Nithsdale, Scotland found a 58% prevalence rate of cigarette smoking, to compare with 28% in the general population. An older study found that as much as 88% of outpatients with schizophrenia were smokers.

Despite the higher prevalence of tobacco smoking, people diagnosed with schizophrenia have a much lower than average chance of developing and dying from lung cancer. While the reason for this is unknown, it may be because of a genetic resistance to the cancer, a side effect of drugs being taken, or a statistical effect of increased likelihood of dying from causes other than lung cancer.

A 2003 study of over 50,000 Swedish conscripts found that there was a small but significant protective effect of smoking cigarettes on the risk of developing schizophrenia later in life. While the authors of the study stressed that the risks of smoking far outweigh these minor benefits, this study provides further evidence for the 'self-medication' theory of smoking in schizophrenia and may give clues as to how schizophrenia might develop at the molecular level. Furthermore, many people with schizophrenia have smoked tobacco products long before they are diagnosed with the illness, and a cohort study of Israeli conscripts found that healthy adolescent smokers were more likely to develop schizophrenia in the future than their nonsmoking peers.

It is of interest that cigarette smoking affects liver function such that the antipsychotic drugs used to treat schizophrenia are broken down in the blood stream more quickly. This means that smokers with schizophrenia need slightly higher doses of antipsychotic drugs in order for them to be effective than do their non-smoking counterparts.

The increased rate of smoking in schizophrenia may be due to a desire to self-medicate with nicotine. One possible reason is that smoking produces a short term effect to improve alertness and cognitive functioning in persons who suffer this illness. It has been postulated that the mechanism of this effect is that people with schizophrenia have a disturbance of nicotinic receptor functioning which is temporarily abated by tobacco use. However, some researchers have questioned whether self-medication is really the best explanation for the association.

A study from 1989 and a 2004 case study show that when haloperidol is administered, nicotine limits the extent to which the antipsychotic increases the sensitivity of the dopamine 2 receptor. Dependent on the dopamine system, symptoms of Tardive Dyskinesia are not found in the nicotine administered patients despite a roughly 70% increase in dopamine receptor activity, but the controls have more than 90% and do develop symptoms. A 1997 study showed that akathisia was significantly reduced upon administration of nicotine when the akathisia was induced by antipsychotics. This gives credence to the idea tobacco could be used to self-medicate by limiting effects of the illness, the medication, or both.

Life Experiences

Social Adversity

The chance of developing schizophrenia has been found to increase with the number of adverse social factors (e.g. indicators of socioeconomic disadvantage or social exclusion) present in childhood. Stressful life events generally precede the onset of schizophrenia. A personal or recent family history of migration is a considerable risk factor for schizophrenia, which has been linked to psychosocial adversity, social defeat from being an outsider, racial discrimination, family dysfunction, unemployment, and poor housing conditions. Unemployment and early separation from parents are some important factors which are responsible for the higher rates of schizophrenia among British African Caribbean populations, in comparison to native African Caribbean populations. This is an example which shows that social disadvantage plays an equally major hand in the onset of schizophrenia as genetics.

Childhood experiences of abuse or trauma are risk factors for a diagnosis of schizophrenia later in life. Recent large-scale general population studies indicate the relationship is a causal one, with an increasing risk with additional experiences of maltreatment, although a critical review suggests conceptual and methodological issues require further research. There is some evidence that adversities may lead to cognitive biases and altered dopamine neurotransmission, a process that has been termed "sensitization". Childhood trauma, and bereavement or separation in families, have been found to be risk factors for schizophrenia and psychosis.

Specific social experiences have been linked to specific psychological mechanisms and psychotic experiences in schizophrenia. In addition, structural neuroimaging studies of victims of sexual abuse and other traumas have sometimes reported findings similar to those sometimes found in psychotic patients, such as thinning of the corpus callosum, loss of volume in the anterior cingulate cortex, and reduced hippocampal volume.

Urbanicity

A particularly stable and replicable finding has been the association between living in an urban environment and the development of schizophrenia, even after factors such as drug use, ethnic group and size of social group have been controlled for. A recent study of 4.4 million men and women in Sweden found a 68%–77% increased risk of diagnosed psychosis for people living in the most urbanized environments, a significant proportion of which is likely to be described as schizophrenia.

The effect does not appear to be due to a higher incidence of obstetric complications in urban environments. The risk increases with the number of years and degree of urban living in childhood and adolescence, suggesting that constant, cumulative, or repeated exposures during upbringing occurring more frequently in urbanized areas are responsible for the association.

Various possible explanations for the effect have been judged unlikely based on the nature of the findings, including infectious causes or a generic stress effect. It is thought to interact with genetic dispositions and, since there appears to be nonrandom variation even across different neighborhoods, and an independent association with social isolation, it has been proposed that the degree of "social capital" (e.g. degree of mutual trust, bonding and safety in neighborhoods) can exert a developmental impact on children growing up in these environments.

Close Relationships

Evidence is consistent that negative attitudes from others increase the risk of schizophrenia relapse, in particular critical comments, hostility, authoritarian, and intrusive or controlling attitudes (termed 'high expressed emotion' by researchers). Although family members and significant others are not held responsible for schizophrenia - the attitudes, behaviors and interactions of all parties are addressed - unsupportive dysfunctional relationships may also contribute to an increased risk of developing schizophrenia. The risk of developing schizophrenia can also be increased by an individual developing a very low sense of self, in which one's boundaries become confused with that of the mother and/ or father. Firm psychological boundaries should be established between one's self and one's identity and one's parents. Pushing the role of parents into the background and developing a healthy sense of self can be a method for recovery. Social support systems are very important for schizophrenics and the people with whom they are in relationships. Recovery from schizophrenia is possible when one develops a healthy self and establishes firm psychological boundaries with each of their parents.

Synergistic Effects

Experiments on mice have provided evidence that several stressors can act together to increase the risk of schizophrenia. In particular, the combination of a maternal infection during pregnancy followed by heightened stress at the onset of sexual maturity markedly increases the probability that a mouse develops symptoms of schizophrenia, whereas the occurrence of one of these factors without the other does not.

Other Views

Schizophrenia is suggested to be a brain disorder rather than a mental illness. It is labeled as a mental illness because the symptoms align as such and the causes of the disorder are not completely known and understood. Psychiatrists R. D. Laing, Silvano Arieti, Theodore Lidz and others have argued that the symptoms of what is called mental illness are comprehensible reactions to impossible demands that society and particularly family life places on some sensitive individuals. Laing, Arieti and Lidz were notable in valuing the *content* of psychotic experience as worthy of interpretation, rather than considering it simply as a secondary and essentially meaningless marker of underlying psychological or neurological distress. Laing described eleven case studies of people diagnosed with schizophrenia and argued that the content of their actions and statements was meaningful and logical in the context of their family and life situations.

In 1956, Gregory Bateson and his colleagues Paul Watzlawick, Donald Jackson, and Jay Haley articulated a theory of schizophrenia, related to Laing's work, as stemming from double bind situations where a person receives different or contradictory messages. Madness was therefore an expression of this distress and should be valued as a cathartic and transformative experience. In the books *Schizophrenia and the Family* and *The Origin and Treatment of Schizophrenic Disorders* Lidz and his colleagues explain their belief that parental behaviour can result in mental illness in children. Arieti's *Interpretation of Schizophrenia* won the 1975 scientific National Book Award in the United States.

The concept of schizophrenia as a result of civilization has been developed further by psychologist Julian Jaynes in his 1976 book *The Origin of Consciousness in the Breakdown of the Bicameral Mind*; he proposed that until the beginning of historic times, schizophrenia or a similar condition was the normal state of human consciousness. This would take the form of a "bicameral mind" where a normal state of low affect, suitable for routine activities, would be interrupted in moments of crisis by "mysterious voices" giving instructions, which early people characterized as interventions from the gods. Researchers into shamanism have speculated that in some cultures schizophrenia or related conditions (such as schizotypal personality disorder) may predispose an individual to becoming a shaman; the experience of having access to multiple realities is not uncommon in schizophrenia, and is a core experience in many shamanic traditions. Equally, the shaman may have the skill to bring on and direct some of the altered states of consciousness psychiatrists label as illness. Psychohistorians, on the other hand, accept the psychiatric diagnoses. However, unlike the current medical model of mental disorders they may argue that poor parenting in tribal societies causes the shaman's schizoid personalities. Commentators such as Paul Kurtz and others have endorsed the idea that major religious figures experienced psychosis, heard voices and displayed delusions of grandeur.

Modern clinical psychological research has indicated a number of processes which may cause or bring on episodes of schizophrenia.

A number of cognitive biases and deficits have been identified. These include attribution biases in social situations, difficulty distinguishing inner speech from speech from an external source (source monitoring), difficulty in adjusting speech to the needs of the hearer, difficulties in the very earliest stages of processing visual information (including reduced latent inhibition), and an attentional bias towards threats.

Some of these tendencies have been shown to worsen or appear when under emotional stress or in confusing situations. As with related neurological findings, they are not shown by all individuals with a diagnosis of schizophrenia, and it is not clear how specific they are to schizophrenia. However, the findings regarding cognitive difficulties in schizophrenia are reliable and consistent enough for some researchers to argue that they are diagnostic.

Impaired capacity to appreciate one's own and others' mental states has been reported to be the single-best predictor of poor social competence in schizophrenia, and similar cognitive features have been identified in close relatives of people diagnosed with schizophrenia.

A number of emotional factors have been implicated in schizophrenia, with some models putting them at the core of the disorder. It was thought that the appearance of blunted affect meant that sufferers did not experience strong emotions, but more recent studies indicate there is often a normal or even heightened level of emotionality, particularly in response to negative events or stressful social situations. Some theories suggest positive symptoms of schizophrenia can result from or be worsened by negative emotions, including depressed feelings and low self-esteem and feelings of vulnerability, inferiority or loneliness. Chronic negative feelings and maladaptive coping skills may explain some of the association between psychosocial stressors and symptomology. Critical and controlling behaviour by significant others (high expressed emotion) causes increased emotional arousal and lowered self-esteem and a subsequent increase in positive symptoms such as unusual thoughts. Countries or cultures where schizotypal personalities or schizophrenia symptoms are more accepted or valued appear to be associated with reduced onset of, or increased recovery from, schizophrenia.

Related studies suggest that the content of delusional and psychotic beliefs in schizophrenia can be meaningful and play a causal or mediating role in reflecting the life history, or social circumstances of the individual. Holding minority socio-cultural beliefs, for example due to ethnic background, has been linked to increased diagnosis of schizophrenia. The way an individual interprets his or her delusions and hallucinations (e.g. as threatening or as potentially positive) has also been found to influence functioning and recovery.

Some experts think autonomy vs intimacy is a motivation for schizophrenic symptoms.

Other lines of work relating to the self in schizophrenia have linked it to psychological dissociation or abnormal states of awareness and identity as understood from phenomenological, such as in self-disorders, and other perspectives.

Psychiatrist Tim Crow has argued that schizophrenia may be the evolutionary price we pay for a left brain hemisphere specialization for language. Since psychosis is associated with greater levels of right brain hemisphere activation and a reduction in the usual left brain hemisphere dominance, our language abilities may have evolved at the cost of causing schizophrenia when this system breaks down.

In alternative medicine, some practitioners believe that there are a vast number of physical causes of what ends up being diagnosed as schizophrenia. While some of these explanations may stretch credulity, others (such as heavy metal poisoning and nutritional imbalances) have been supported at least somewhat by research. However, it is not entirely clear how many (if any) patients initially diagnosed with schizophrenia these alternative explanations may account for.

Psychological stress may worsen schizophrenia.

Management of Schizophrenia

Management of schizophrenia usually involved many aspects including psychological, pharmacological, social, educational, and employment-related interventions directed to recovery, reducing the impact of the disease on quality of life, social functioning, and longevity.

Hospitalization

Hospitalization may occur with severe episodes of schizophrenia. This can be voluntary or (if mental health legislation allows it) involuntary (called civil or involuntary commitment).

Long-term inpatient stays are now less common due to deinstitutionalization, although still occur. Following (or in lieu of) a hospital admission, support services available can include drop-in centers, visits from members of a community mental health team or Assertive Community Treatment team, supported employment and patient-led support groups. Efforts to avoid repeated hospitalization include the obtaining of community treatment orders which,following judicial approval, coerce the affected individual to receive psychiatric treatment including long-acting injections of anti-psychotic medication. This legal mechanism has been shown to increase the affected patient's time out of the hospital.

Medication

The mainstay of psychiatric treatment for schizophrenia is antipsychotic medication. Medication might improve a number of outcomes found to be important to patients, including positive, acute and psychotic symptoms, and social and vocational functioning. Medication can reduce the "positive" symptoms of psychosis. Most antipsychotics are thought to take around 7 to 14 days to have their main effect. However, these drugs fail to significantly ameliorate the negative symptoms and cognitive dysfunction. There is evidence of clozapine, amisulpride, olanzapine and risperidone being the most effective medications, although a high proportion of studies of risperidone were undertaken by its manufacturer, Janssen-Cilag, and should be interpreted with this in mind. In those on antipsychotics, continued use decreases the risk of relapse. There is little evidence regarding consistent benefits from their use beyond two or three years.

Treatment of schizophrenia changed dramatically in the mid-1950s with the development and introduction of the first antipsychotic chlorpromazine. Others such as haloperidol and trifluoperazine soon followed.

It remains unclear whether the newer antipsychotics reduce the chances of developing neuroleptic malignant syndrome, a rare but serious and potentially fatal neurological disorder most often caused by an adverse reaction to neuroleptic or antipsychotic drugs.

Most people on antipsychotics get side effects. People on typical antipsychotics tend to have a higher rate of extrapyramidal side effects while some atypicals are associated with considerable weight gain, diabetes and risk of metabolic syndrome; this is most pronounced with olanzapine, while risperidone and quetiapine are also associated with weight gain. Risperidone has a similar rate of extrapyramidal symptoms to haloperidol. The American Psychiatric Association generally recommends that atypicals be used as first line treatment in most patients, but further states that therapy should be individually optimized for each patient.

Response of symptoms to medication is variable; "Treatment-resistant schizophrenia" is the failure to respond to two or more antipsychotic medications given in therapeutic doses for six weeks or more. Patients in this category may be prescribed clozapine, a medication of superior effectiveness but several potentially lethal side effects including agranulocytosis and myocarditis. Clozapine is the only medication proven to be more effective for persons who do not respond to other types of antipsychotics. It also appears to reduce suicide in people with schizophrenia. As clozapine suppresses the development of bone marrow, in turn reducing white blood cells which can lead to infection, blood tests are taken for the first six months on this medication. A update to the existing Cochrane review was done in 2009; which showed that clozapine though effective, has its own adverse(dangerous) effects in the form of decline in white blood cell count seen frequently in children,and adolescents. The effectiveness in the studies also needs to be interpreted with caution as the studies may have an increased risk of bias.

Psychosocial

Psychotherapy is also widely recommended, though not widely used in the treatment of schizophrenia, due to reimbursement problems or lack of training. As a result, treatment is often confined to psychiatric medication.

Cognitive behavioral therapy (CBT) is used to target specific symptoms and improve related issues such as self-esteem and social functioning. Although the results of early trials were inconclusive as the therapy advanced from its initial applications in the mid-1990s, meta-analytic reviews suggested CBT to be an effective treatment for the psychotic symptoms of schizophrenia. Nonetheless more recent meta analyses have cast doubt upon the utility of CBT as a treatment for the symptoms of psychosis.

Another approach is cognitive remediation therapy, a technique aimed at remediating the neurocognitive deficits sometimes present in schizophrenia. Based on techniques of neuropsychological rehabilitation, early evidence has shown it to be cognitively effective, resulting in the improvement of previous deficits in psychomotor speed, verbal memory, nonverbal memory, and executive function, such improvements being related to measurable changes in brain activation as measured by fMRI.

Metacognitive training: In view of many empirical findings suggesting deficits of metacognition (thinking about one's thinking, reflecting upon one's cognitive process) in patients with schizophrenia, metacognitive training (MCT) is increasingly adopted as a complementary treatment approach. MCT aims at sharpening the awareness of patients for a variety of cognitive biases (e.g. jumping to conclusions, attributional biases, over-confidence in errors), which are implicated in the formation and maintenance of schizophrenia positive symptoms (especially delusions), and to ultimately replace these biases with functional cognitive strategies.

The training consists of 8 modules and can be obtained cost-free from the internet in 15 languages. Studies confirm the feasibility and lend preliminary support to the efficacy of the intervention. Recently, an individualized format has been developed which combines the metacognitive approach with methods derived from cognitive-behavioral therapy.

Family Therapy or Education, which addresses the whole family system of an individual with a diagnosis of schizophrenia, has been consistently found to be beneficial, at least if the duration of intervention is longer-term. Aside from therapy, the impact of schizophrenia on families and the burden on careers has been recognized, with the increasing availability of self-help books on the subject. There is also some evidence for benefits from social skills training, although there have also been significant negative findings. Some studies have explored the possible benefits of music therapy and other creative therapies.

The Soteria model is alternative to inpatient hospitalization using full non professional care and a minimal medication approach. Although evidence is limited, a review found the programme equally as effective as treatment with medications but due to the limited evidence did not recommend it as a standard treatment. Training in the detection of suble facial expressions has been used to improve facial emotional recognition.

Diet

An unconventional approach is the use of omega-3 fatty acids, with one study finding some benefits from their use as a dietary supplement.

A 2003 review of four randomized controlled trials of EPA (an omega-3 fatty acid) vs. placebo as adjunctive treatment for schizophrenia found that two of the trials detected a significant improvement on positive and negative symptoms, and suggested that EPA may be an effective adjunct to antipsychotics. The most recent meta-analysis (2006) failed however to find a significant effect. A 2007 review found that studies of omega-3 fatty acids in schizophrenia, despite being mostly of high quality, have produced inconsistent results and small effect sizes of doubtful clinical significance. Individualized nutrition interventions and supplementation has been proposed as an adjunct to pharmacological therapy in people with schizophrenia, though this approach has not been evaluated in clinical trials to determine the efficacy of such an approach in improving symptoms.

Other

Transcranial magnetic stimulation (TMS) appears to be effecting in alleviating the negative symptoms and cognitive deficits see in schizophrenia, a recent double-blind randomized sham controlled study of deep-TMS add-on treatment noted an 8-point reduction in the Scale for the Assessment of Negative Symptoms (SANS) in patients.

Electroconvulsive therapy is not considered a first line treatment but may be prescribed in cases where other treatments have failed. It is more effective where symptoms of catatonia are present, and is recommended for use under NICE guidelines in the UK for catatonia if previously effective, though there is no recommendation for use for schizophrenia otherwise. Psychosurgery has now become a rare procedure and is not a recommended treatment for schizophrenia.

A study in 2014 conducted by an Australian researcher indicated that the pericarp powder of *Garcinia mangostana L.* have the ability to reduce oxidative stress as an effective treatment for schizophrenia by increasing glutathione S-transferase levels which enhances mitochondrial activity over a period of 180 days under a sustained intake of 1000 mg/day.

References

- Sciacca, Kathleen; Thompson, Christina M. (Summer 1996). "Program Development and Integrated Treatment Across Systems for Dual Diagnosis: Mental Illness, Drug Addiction And Alcoholism, MIDAA". Journal of Mental Health Administration. 23 (3): 288–297
- Evans, Katie; Sullivan, Michael J. (1 March 2001). Dual Diagnosis: Counseling the Mentally Ill Substance Abuser (2nd ed.). Guilford Press. pp. 75–76. ISBN 978-1-57230-446-8
- "Report to Congress on the prevention and treatment of co-occurring substance abuse disorders and mental disorders". SAMHSA. November 2001. Retrieved 1 May 2012
- Barrera A, McKenna PJ, Berrios GE (2009). "Formal thought disorder, neuropsychology and insight in schizophrenia". Psychopathology. 42 (4): 264–9. PMID 19521143. doi:10.1159/000224150
- Elliott A.; Mahmood T.; Smalligan R. D. (2012). "Cocaine Bugs: A Case Report of Cocaine-Induced Delusions of Parasitosis". The American Journal on Addictions. 21: 180–181. doi:10.1111/j.1521-0391.2011.00208.x
- Alan F. Schatzberg; Charles B. Nemeroff (2009). The American Psychiatric Publishing Textbook of Psychopharmacology. The American Psychiatric Publishing. pp. 847–48. ISBN 978-1-58562-309-9
- American Psychiatric Association (2006). "Practice Guidelines for the Treatment of Patients with Substance Use Disorders, 2nd ed". Retrieved 5 April 2013
- Mueser KT; Drake RE; Wallach MA (1998). "Dual diagnosis: a review of etiological theories". Addictive Behaviors. 23 (6): 717–34. PMID 9801712. doi:10.1016/S0306-4603(98)00073-2
- Broderick, P.; Benjamin, A. B. (2004). "Caffeine and psychiatric symptoms: A review". The Journal of the Oklahoma State Medical Association. 97 (12): 538–542. PMID 15732884
- Jones, Daniel (2003) [1917], Peter Roach, James Hartmann and Jane Setter, eds., English Pronouncing Dictionary, Cambridge: Cambridge University Press, ISBN 3-12-539683-2
- Kendler, K.S.; Parnas, J. (2012). Philosophical Issues in Psychiatry II: Nosology. International Perspectives in Philosophy & Psychiatry. OUP Oxford. pp. 242–243. ISBN 978-0-19-964220-5. Retrieved 2016-04-12
- DiSCLAFANI; et al. (1981). "Drug-induced psychosis: Emergency diagnosis and management". Psychosomatics. 22 (10): 845–855. doi:10.1016/s0033-3182(81)73092-5
- Mazure CM, Bowers MB (1 February 1998). "Pretreatment plasma HVA predicts neuroleptic response in manic psychosis". Journal of Affective Disorders. 48 (1): 83–6. PMID 9495606. doi:10.1016/S0165-0327(97)00159-6
- Sims, Andrew (2002). Symptoms in the mind: an introduction to descriptive psychopathology. Philadelphia: W. B. Saunders. p. 127. ISBN 0-7020-2627-1
- McNeill, Ann (2001). "Smoking and mental health — a review of the literature" (PDF). SmokeFree London Programme. Archived from the original (PDF) on 2006-09-24. Retrieved 2006-12-14
- Tsuang MT, Stone WS, Faraone SV. Toward reformulating the diagnosis of schizophrenia. American Journal of Psychiatry. 2000;157(7):1041–50. doi:10.1176/appi.ajp.157.7.1041. PMID 10873908

- Newman, Barbara M.; Newman, Philip R. (2011). “Isolation”. Development Through Life: A Psychosocial Approach. Wadsworth. p. 469. ISBN 978-1-111-34466-5
- Compton, Michael T. (2005-11-16). “Cigarette Smoking in Individuals with Schizophrenia”. Medscape Psychiatry & Mental Health. Retrieved 2007-05-17
- Joyce, E. (2005). “Origins of cognitive dysfunction in schizophrenia: Clues from age at onset”. The British Journal of Psychiatry. 186 (2): 93–95. PMID 15684229. doi:10.1192/bjp.186.2.93
- Jaynes J (1976). The origin of consciousness in the breakdown of the bicameral mind. Boston: Houghton Mifflin. ISBN 0-395-20729-0
- “Getting crowded on chromosome 11q22—make way for phosphohippolin”. Schizophrenia Research Forum. 14 March 2007. Archived from the original on 2007-04-30. Retrieved 2007-05-16
- Frodl, T. (Sep 2010). “Comorbidity of ADHD and Substance Use Disorder (SUD): a neuroimaging perspective.”. J Atten Disord. 14 (2): 109–20. PMID 20495160. doi:10.1177/1087054710365054

Permissions

All chapters in this book are published with permission under the Creative Commons Attribution Share Alike License or equivalent. Every chapter published in this book has been scrutinized by our experts. Their significance has been extensively debated. The topics covered herein carry significant information for a comprehensive understanding. They may even be implemented as practical applications or may be referred to as a beginning point for further studies.

We would like to thank the editorial team for lending their expertise to make the book truly unique. They have played a crucial role in the development of this book. Without their invaluable contributions this book wouldn't have been possible. They have made vital efforts to compile up to date information on the varied aspects of this subject to make this book a valuable addition to the collection of many professionals and students.

This book was conceptualized with the vision of imparting up-to-date and integrated information in this field. To ensure the same, a matchless editorial board was set up. Every individual on the board went through rigorous rounds of assessment to prove their worth. After which they invested a large part of their time researching and compiling the most relevant data for our readers.

The editorial board has been involved in producing this book since its inception. They have spent rigorous hours researching and exploring the diverse topics which have resulted in the successful publishing of this book. They have passed on their knowledge of decades through this book. To expedite this challenging task, the publisher supported the team at every step. A small team of assistant editors was also appointed to further simplify the editing procedure and attain best results for the readers.

Apart from the editorial board, the designing team has also invested a significant amount of their time in understanding the subject and creating the most relevant covers. They scrutinized every image to scout for the most suitable representation of the subject and create an appropriate cover for the book.

The publishing team has been an ardent support to the editorial, designing and production team. Their endless efforts to recruit the best for this project, has resulted in the accomplishment of this book. They are a veteran in the field of academics and their pool of knowledge is as vast as their experience in printing. Their expertise and guidance has proved useful at every step. Their uncompromising quality standards have made this book an exceptional effort. Their encouragement from time to time has been an inspiration for everyone.

The publisher and the editorial board hope that this book will prove to be a valuable piece of knowledge for students, practitioners and scholars across the globe.

Index

A

Abdominal Epilepsy, 25-26

Absence Seizure, 3, 89, 105-106, 108

Altered Signalling Cascades, 170

Alternative Medicine, 14, 225

Anti-epileptic Drugs, 20, 35-36, 45, 70

Antipsychotic Medication, 125, 132, 135-136, 155, 159, 161, 174-175, 187, 206, 218

Atonic Seizures, 3, 13, 33, 35, 90, 93, 98, 100, 117

B

Barbiturates, 95, 114, 121

Benign Infantile Epilepsy, 72

Benign Myoclonic Epilepsy, 26

Benzodiazepines, 12, 95, 118, 120-121, 135, 184, 186

C

Carbamazepine, 13, 21, 32, 43, 56, 65-66, 83, 108, 121

Catamenial Epilepsy, 74-77, 88

Clonic Seizures, 3, 15, 17, 20, 22, 27-29, 33-35, 39, 46, 57, 78-79, 82, 90, 98-100, 110, 112, 115-116

Cognitive Dysfunction, 10, 127, 226, 230

Complex Focal Seizure, 102, 104

Contraindicated Drugs, 108

Cyclic Progesterone Therapy, 78

D

Dementia Praecox, 140, 143-145, 155, 213

Diaphragmatic Flutter, 111

Disorganized Schizophrenia, 156

Dopamine Dysfunction, 161

Dual Diagnosis, 185-186, 188, 229

E

Economic Costs, 18, 97

Electroencephalogram, 1, 6, 10, 26, 84-85, 89, 96, 110, 118, 158

Epidemiology, 16, 21, 29, 54, 68, 80, 83, 96, 122, 138, 159, 208, 214

Epilepsia Partialis Continua, 101, 122-123

Estrogen, 74-77, 209

F

Febrile Seizures Plus, 26, 29

Fluorescent Lighting, 58

Focal Seizures, 2-3, 5-6, 8, 11, 13, 15, 36, 80, 82, 89-90, 93-94, 101-102

Fosphenytoin, 121

G

Gabapentin, 13, 43, 56, 66, 83, 106, 108, 113

Generalized Seizures, 2-3, 6, 13, 15, 19, 29, 35, 62, 89-90, 93, 98-101, 108, 115

Glutamate Abnormalities, 162

H

Hallucinations, 37-38, 47, 103, 126-127, 133-135, 147, 152-154, 156-157, 161, 166, 171, 173, 189-191, 193, 204-207, 217-218, 225

Head Injuries, 11, 63

I

Idiopathic Generalized Epilepsy, 26, 28-29

Immune System Abnormalities, 163

Immune System Hypothesis, 149

Inexplicable Feelings, 102

Inhibitory Transmission, 170

Interneuron Dysfunction, 162-163

J

Jacksonian March, 3, 90, 103, 122

L

Landau-kleffner Syndrome, 83-84, 88

Lennox-gastaut Syndrome, 8, 10, 110, 117

Lethargy, 105, 157

Luteal Classification, 76

M

Mental Functioning, 50, 70

Metabolic Abnormalities, 71

Middle Ear Myoclonus, 112

Myelination Abnormalities, 163

Myoclonic Epilepsy, 26-27, 29, 32-33, 35, 69-70, 78, 107, 110, 113, 124

Myoclonic Seizures, 3, 13, 27, 33, 35, 78, 98-100, 109
Myoclonus, 69-71, 78-79, 81-82, 99-100, 108-115, 118, 121-122, 124

N
Nature Of Trauma, 63
Nervous System Disorder, 71
Neurological Disorder, 45, 137, 226
Neuronal Ceroid Lipofuscinoses, 79
Nonconvulsive Status Epilepticus, 119

O
Obsessive-compulsive Disorder (OCD), 4, 206
Oxidative Stress, 161, 163-164, 229

P
Palatal Myoclonus, 112
Paranoid Schizophrenia, 133, 152-156
Partial Seizures, 35-39, 45-46, 54, 62, 94, 97-99, 101-104, 108, 118-119, 124
Pathophysiology, 30, 42, 74, 88, 115, 160-163
Pediatric Schizophrenia, 157
Perimenstrual Classification, 76
Phenytoin, 12-13, 18, 26, 43, 53, 56, 65-66, 79, 83, 95, 114, 118, 120-121
Photosensitive Epilepsy, 17, 56, 59-60
Pinball Machines, 58
Post-traumatic Epilepsy, 25, 61, 92
Post-traumatic Seizures, 61, 63, 68, 92
Postictal Period, 3, 39, 91
Preserved Consciousness, 102
Progesterone, 74-78, 88
Prognosis, 8, 15, 28, 33-34, 39, 60, 67, 83, 87,
96, 101, 115, 122, 154, 156, 159
Progressive Myoclonus Epilepsy, 70, 78, 110
Psychological Well-being, 4
Psychosocial Interventions, 137
Psychotic Symptoms, 103, 128, 132-135, 139, 157, 160-161, 174, 190, 205-206, 208, 226-227

R
Ragged Red Fibres, 79
Rolandic Epilepsy, 10, 80, 82-83, 88

S
Schizophrenia, 85, 99, 125-182, 184, 188-196, 198-202, 204-230 Seizures, 1-11, 13-23, 26-30, 33-43, 45-48, 50-74, 77-84, 87-113, 115-124
Self-domestication Hypothesis, 149
Severity of Trauma, 63
Shamanistic Hypothesis, 148
Social Advantage Hypothesis, 148
Social Brain Hypothesis, 147
Social Withdrawal, 128, 135, 147, 157
Status Epilepticus, 12, 15, 19, 64, 82, 84, 86, 90, 95-96, 100-101, 108, 117-122, 124
Substance Use, 137, 179, 183-186, 218, 229
Synaptic Pruning, 168

T
Tonic-clonic Seizure, 3, 12, 89, 100, 102, 105, 115-116
Type I Sialidosis, 79-80

U
Unprovoked Seizures, 7, 62
Unverricht-lundborg Disease, 70, 79

V
Valproate, 13, 43, 56, 60, 66, 83, 106, 108, 114-115, 121
Video Games, 14, 58-59

W
Web Design, 59